Essential Surgical Skills

2nd Edition

David A. Sherris, M.D.

Associate Professor and Interim Chair of Otolaryngology,
University at Buffalo, State University of New York, Buffalo, New York;
Former Associate Professor and Chair
Division of Facial Plastic Surgery,
Department of Otorhinolaryngology,
Mayo Clinic, Rochester, Minnesota

Eugene B. Kern, M.D.

Emeritus Endicott Professor of Medicine, Mayo Foundation,
Emeritus Professor of Rhinology and Facial Plastic Surgery,
Division of Facial Plastic Surgery,
Department of Otorhinolaryngology,
Mayo Clinic, Rochester, Minnesota

KT-405-135

SAUNDERS

An Imprint of Elsevier

SAUNDERS

An Imprint of Elsevier

The Curtis Center
Independence Square West
Philadelphia, Pennsylvania 19106

Essential Surgical Skills 2nd Edition　　　　　　　　　　　　　　ISBN 0-7216-3950-x

---

NOTICE

Care has been taken to confirm the accuracy of the information presented and to describe gener-
ally accepted practices. However, the authors, editor, and publisher are not responsible for errors
or omissions or for any consequences from application of the information in this book and make
no warranty, express or implied, with respect to the contents of the publication.

The authors, editor, and publisher have exerted efforts to ensure that medical equipment and
devices, drug selection and dosage set forth in this text are in accordance with current recom-
mendations and practice at the time of publication. However, in view of ongoing research,
changes in government regulations, and the constant flow of information relating to medical
therapy and drug reactions, the reader is urged to check the package insert for each medical
device and drug for any change in indications and dosage and for added warnings and precau-
tions. This is particularly important when the recommended agent is a new or infrequently
employed drug.

Some drugs and medical devices presented in this publication have Food and Drug
Administration (FDA) clearance for limited use in restricted research settings. It is the responsi-
bility of the health care providers to ascertain the FDA status of each drug or device planned for
use in their clinical practice.

Printed in the United States of America
Last digit is the print number　9　8　7　6　5　4　3　2

Dedication

To our families
for their support

To our teachers
for their wisdom

To our students
for their direction

To our patients
for their trust

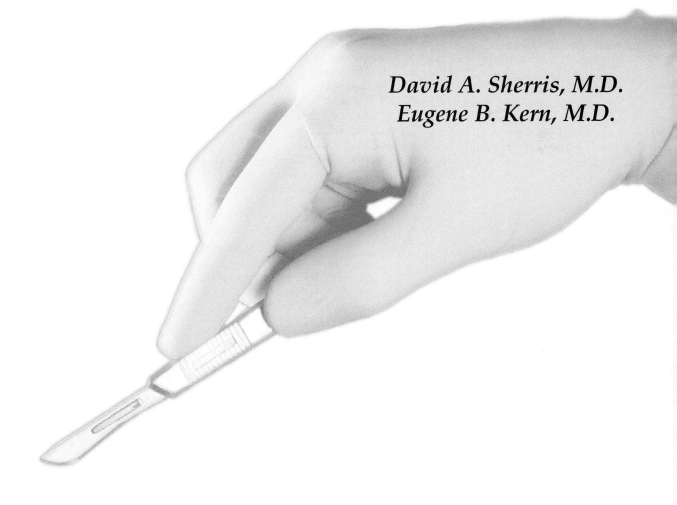

David A. Sherris, M.D.
Eugene B. Kern, M.D.

Table of Contents

**CD-ROM icon indicates supplemental audio-visual
materials that can be seen and heard on the CD.**

Preface to First Edition

The current education for medical students in the realm of surgery has been markedly compacted; often the allotted time in which the principles of surgery must be taught and learned does not extend beyond six weeks. This adverse situation is compounded by the reduced time that the surgical faculty spends with students. The same socioeconomic forces that have caused this behavior pattern also account for the reduction of time during which the surgical faculty formally educates. Sadly, basic principles have been poorly addressed. Residency Review Committees concerned with this circumstance have mandated exposure of surgical residents to basic science as it pertains to surgery. This is certainly appropriate but it is equally appropriate to stress basic technical principles of operative procedures because the technical therapies are uniquely in the surgeon's armamentarium. The ability to treat by an operation distinguishes the surgeon from the physician.

In learning the principles of surgery, the principles of technique constitute an essential ingredient. This ingredient has been neglected recently. The authors of Basic Surgical Skills have filled a void. They have provided in a succinct, readable, and understandable text the basics of surgical techniques. The CD-ROM elegantly clarifies the written words. The audience should include all medical students as they rotate through their exposure to surgery and all residents in surgical specialties as they launch their training programs. The word "education" derives from the Latin, meaning "lead out." The combined words and views serve to lead the novitiates in the field of surgery into the surgical arena, the operating room. ∎

Seymour I. Schwartz, M.D., F.A.C.S.*

Professor of Surgery

University of Rochester School of Medicine and Dentistry

Rochester, New York

* F.A.C.S. - Fellow, American College of Surgeons, past president of the American College of Surgeons

Preface to Second Edition

*T*he curriculum of today's medical schools has expanded greatly during the past few decades, and the cognitive knowledge that students are required to master has increased proportionately. Many of the traditional medical sciences, such as anatomy and physiology, by necessity have been relegated to a few short months to accommodate this new knowledge. Many traditional disciplines also now center on body systems and are taught concomitantly. Surgery, too, has expanded in recent years, and no longer is it possible for the student to focus on a specific career choice. Instead, today's primary emphasis is on the broad principles of surgery, and then only in a markedly condensed fashion. For those students interested in a surgical career, exposure to both surgical faculty and a surgical skills laboratory is limited, with the end result that most medical schools no longer teach surgical technique.

Aimed toward the novice, Essential Surgical Skills corrects this deficiency. The authors have greatly enhanced this second edition through constructive feedback from past users of their first edition. Original sections have been enlarged and new sections, such as endoscopy, added. Suture, Needles and Knots has been completely revised to include illustrations for both right-and left-handed surgeons. Obtaining Hemostasis has been broadened to include topical hemostatic agents, and several simple operations, such as appendectomy and skin flaps, are illustrated. The CD-ROM has been expanded to two volumes. New video and film animation has been added to complement the textbook and are presented in a user-friendly manner. Essential Surgical Skills takes the beginner through every phase of surgical technique and leads the novice from the skills laboratory to the operating room. It should be required reading for all budding surgeons. ∎

Peter C. Pairolero, M.D., F.A.C.S.

Professor and Chair
Department of Surgery
Mayo Medical School
Rochester, Minnesota

Introduction to Second Edition

It has been three years since the first edition of Basic Surgical Skills appeared on October 1, 1999. We have continued to teach our students at Mayo Medical School and at a number of other medical institutions around the country. Although we have been gratified with the 5 star (★★★★★) overall rating from reviewers on line at Amazon.com, we have tried, and hopefully succeeded, in expanding and improving this work. We have changed the title from the elementary *Basic Surgical Skills* to the more inclusive and fundamental *Essential Surgical Skills*.

Through constructive feedback from numerous sources we have modified and enlarged the content without complicating the concepts which are still focused toward a succinct, readable, lavishly illustrated practical book enhanced by the visuals, videos, film animations and narration on the enclosed 2 CD ROM set, though materials have been added that will challenge more advanced students as well. This entire program is still for students. As a student, you must learn the essential technical skills necessary to become a competent surgeon or surgical assistant. We have expanded the knot tying sections to include material for both the right handed and left handed surgeon. The materials are presented in a user-friendly manner. Thus, the surgical scrub, gowning and gloving, anesthetics, infiltration techniques, basic instruments, incisions, wound closures, needles, suture material, suturing techniques, knot tying (right and left handed), basic soft tissue flaps, the fundamentals of tissue injury, hemostasis, coagulation, wound healing and general postoperative care will all be covered in this work. We are adding a section on endoscopic surgery, endoscopic suturing and endoscopic knot tying. We want you to learn to perform the essential maneuvers fundamental to all surgery.

We are not teaching the art, or compassion of medicine or surgery. These arts and the details of judgement of specific surgical problems related to, for example, general, orthopedic, cardiac, or other forms of surgery are just beyond the scope of this work. We have designed the book to be visual and concise to speed the learning process. The text is brief and there are over 500 drawings and photographs. The words that are bold and underlined in the text are defined in the glossary. For example, **surgery** is underlined in the text, so it appears in the glossary. We have designed both CD-ROMs to emphasize the essentials and supplement the manual with exercises in both animated and live filmed video presentations for your study and review. The CD-ROM icon ⊙ indicates supplemental audio-visual materials that can be seen and heard on the CD Disc 1 and Disc 2.

You will practice the surgical techniques on pigs' feet. In addition, there will be tests of your knowledge. Knowledge of surgical ideas and the technical experience gained on pigs' feet will make you self-assured. Being self-assured in the operating room is a great feeling. Lets begin to learn the essential skills so you can stride into the operating room with knowledge, experience and confidence. Others have done it before and you can learn it too!

A. The Operating Room

The operating room is a special and unique place. The personnel are trained for their specific jobs and routines.

Anesthesiologists and **nurse anesthetists** are an important part of the surgical team. They are responsible for the anesthetic care of the surgical patient whether surgery is performed under general **intubation** anesthesia, attended local anesthesia, or local anesthesia.

During general intubation anesthesia, the patient is totally asleep. Under attended local anesthesia, the patient is awake but receiving some type of sedation. Under local anesthesia alone the patient is not sedated, and monitoring is less essential. The vital signs, blood pressure, pulse, **oxygen saturation**, and **electrocardiogram** are all monitored by the anesthesia team. The surgical "scrub" nurse (gowned and gloved in a **sterile** manner) is responsible for the set-up of the surgical instruments. The "scrub" nurse also helps direct the operating room activities in an orderly and efficient manner. The "circulating nurse" is also in attendance. This individual is unscrubbed and unsterile and is helpful in obtaining various materials when needed during the surgery. He/she also assists in taking specimens to **pathology**, answering pagers and telephone calls, and various other activities as they arise during the surgical procedure. The surgeon and surgical assistants are also an integral part of the surgical team.

The operating room atmosphere should be one of professionalism — warm, friendly, caring and efficient. Frequently music is played in order to provide a sense of relaxation to the environment. There are times when a situation in the operating room can be tense. It takes practice and discipline for the many personality types who are in the operating room to maintain their cool during the stress of an operation. Loss of control can be demeaning to the staff in an operating room setting and has no place in the professional surgical environment. There are times, however, when a situation becomes so stressful that control is difficult. Words may be said in frustration or anger. It's never too late to apologize! The entire team is present to help the surgeon and surgical assistants accomplish the task for the welfare of the patient. Maintain your cool, become a teacher, and the golden rule is certainly applicable here. Treat people the way you would like to be treated. It's a great and rare privilege to be involved in the miracle of health restored. The operating room is a place where that miracle frequently unfolds.

B. Anatomy of Skin and Deeper Areas

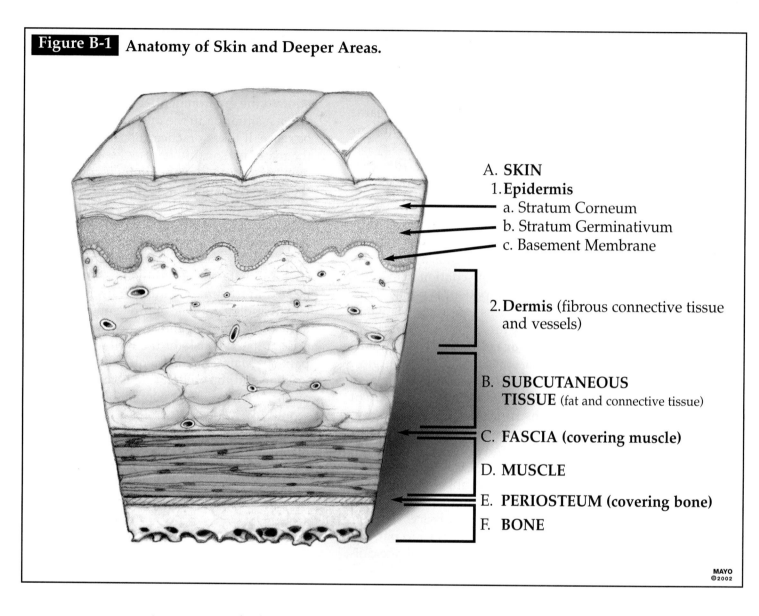

Figure B-1 Anatomy of Skin and Deeper Areas.

A. **SKIN**
  1. **Epidermis**
      a. Stratum Corneum
      b. Stratum Germinativum
      c. Basement Membrane

  2. **Dermis** (fibrous connective tissue and vessels)

B. **SUBCUTANEOUS TISSUE** (fat and connective tissue)

C. **FASCIA (covering muscle)**

D. **MUSCLE**

E. **PERIOSTEUM (covering bone)**

F. **BONE**

MAYO
©2002

Anatomy of Skin and Deeper Areas

The skin is waterproof and serves as a protective barrier for the internal environment. The two layers comprising the skin surface are 1.) epidermis and 2.) dermis **(Figure B-1)**

1.Epidermis has two distinct layers

a. Stratum Corneum
This is the outer (top) keratinized epithelial layer. This outer avascular epithelial layer is insensitive and is continuously being abraded, **sloughed** and regenerated from the deep germinating layer of the epidermis.

b. Stratum Germinativum
This germinating layer produces the new epithelial cells that migrate to the surface and eventually become keratinized and become the new outer (top) layer of skin.

Both the stratum corneum and stratum germinativum are supported by a basement membrane.

B. Anatomy of Skin and Deeper Areas

2. Dermis

This is a dense vascular layer that nourishes the epidermal layers. This layer contains collagen which gives it toughness and strength. Numerous vessels course beneath the dermis in the subdermal plexus, which supplies oxygen and nutrients to the upper layers of skin.

The subdermal plexus is the main blood supply to any surgically created local flaps of the skin. And it is these blood vessels that supply the life sustaining oxygen and nutrition.

3. Deeper Areas

Subcutaneous tissue is composed of connective tissue, nerves, capillaries, veins, lymphatic vessels, adipose (fat) tissue and various glands (sweat and sebaceous).

Fascia is a connective tissue layer that envelops muscle. The periosteum is a dense connective tissue layer attached to the underlying bone and is responsible for supplying the bone with nourishment through its blood supply.

C. The Wound

Figure C-1

Wound (incision)

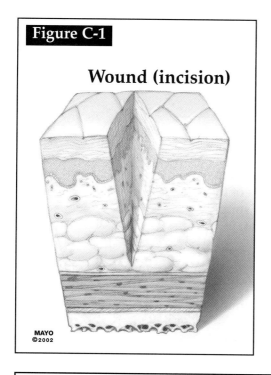

MAYO
©2002

1. Tissue Injury - Wounding

Any break or incision in the epithelial surface, whether the epithelial surface is skin or mucosa is called a wound. **(Figure C-1)** The process of repairing a wound is called healing.

Following a wound (tissue injury) or incision of the skin the body responds by trying to resurface the break in the skin surface. This process is called **re-epithelialization (Figure C-2).** A moist environment facilitates re-epithelialization. Epithelial migration begins within the first few hours of wounding.

Re-epithelialization is an uncomplicated process and occurs rapidly. Tissue injury to the deeper structures requires a more complicated process of repair which follows three distinct phases.

Figure C-2 Re-epithelization - from the Stratum Germinativum

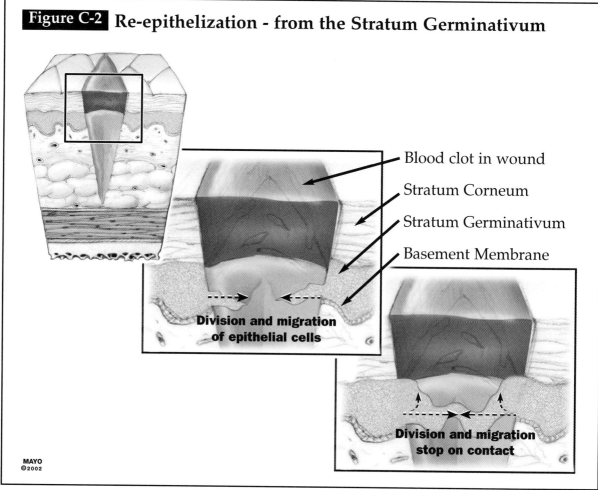

Blood clot in wound

Stratum Corneum

Stratum Germinativum

Basement Membrane

Division and migration of epithelial cells

Division and migration stop on contact

MAYO
©2002

C. The Wound

These three distinct stages of tissue injury (wounding) progress from the first **inflammatory stage** to the second **proliferative stage** to the third and final stage of healing which includes remodeling and **scar maturation stage**. Actually these stages overlap but for purposes of understanding they are neatly divided into three stages. These times are approximate.

- **Stage 1: Inflammation (Vasodilation)** (Day 0 - Day 7)
- **Stage 2: Proliferation** (Day 7 - Day 21)
- **Stage 3: Scar maturation** (Day 21 - 1 year)

a. Stage I, Inflammation (minutes to 7 days)
After the initial tissue injury three reactions occur.

First Reaction - Vasoconstriction
This lasts 5- 10 minutes to reduce blood loss and is followed by vasodilation.

Second Reaction - Vasodilation
Vasodilation increases the blood supply to the wound so oxygen and cellular components can aid wound healing. The increased blood supply causes **erythematous** (red) skin changes. The cellular response includes a white blood cell (**leukocyte)** response. These leukocytes kill bacteria and remove damaged tissue by action of **enzymes**. This removal of injured tissue is termed **debridement**. Pain occurs as a normal protective reaction to tissue injury. These leukocytes from the blood change into macrophages in the tissue which continue to phagocytize (engulf and digest)

bacteria, debris, and dead tissue. These macrophages also secrete substances that stimulate **fibroblasts** to produce **collagen**. Collagen is required for healing and marks entry into the next stage of collagen proliferation. In order for collagen proliferation to proceed, the wound must be free of bacteria, debris and dead tissue. Thus, the need for wound irrigation and debridement (removal) of badly damaged and devitalized tissue by the surgeon is required.

Third Reaction - Coagulation
During injury the coagulation cascade is stimulated and platelets are released forming fibrin plugs and fibrin clots. The fibrin blood clot helps to stop the bleeding. Numerous chemicals are released to signal the beginning of repair and the healing process **(Figure C-3)**.

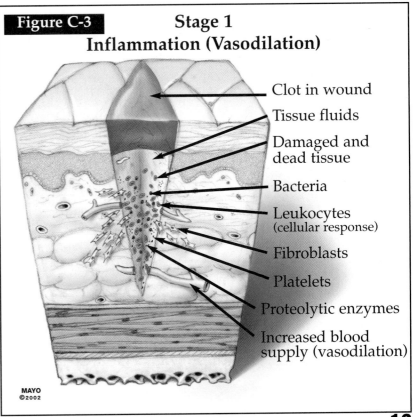

Figure C-3

Stage 1 Inflammation (Vasodilation)

- Clot in wound
- Tissue fluids
- Damaged and dead tissue
- Bacteria
- Leukocytes (cellular response)
- Fibroblasts
- Platelets
- Proteolytic enzymes
- Increased blood supply (vasodilation)

MAYO ©2002

C. The Wound

b. Stage 2, Proliferation (day 7 to day 21)
This stage consists of vascular proliferation and collagen deposition covering the time needed for replacing dead tissue. This begins at about 1 week and lasts about 14 days (day 7 - day 21). The leukocytes, which change to tissue macrophages, stimulate the fibroblasts to produce collagen fibers which are dispensed throughout the wound. These fibroblasts become the predominate cell at about the 5th to 7th day. The macrophages stimulate production of chemicals which causes fibrous tissue and new blood vessel growth. New blood vessels bring oxygen and nutrients to the healing wound. The new, vascular tissue that forms has a granular appearance and is called **granulation tissue.** This granulation tissue is critical for the normal transition from the inflammatory stage to the proliferating stage of wound healing. It is this granulation tissue that fills the gaps of the missing damaged tissue. After this proliferation of granulation tissue and fibroblasts the wound contracts and enters the final stage of wound healing, that of remodeling of collagen and scar maturation **(Figure C-4).**

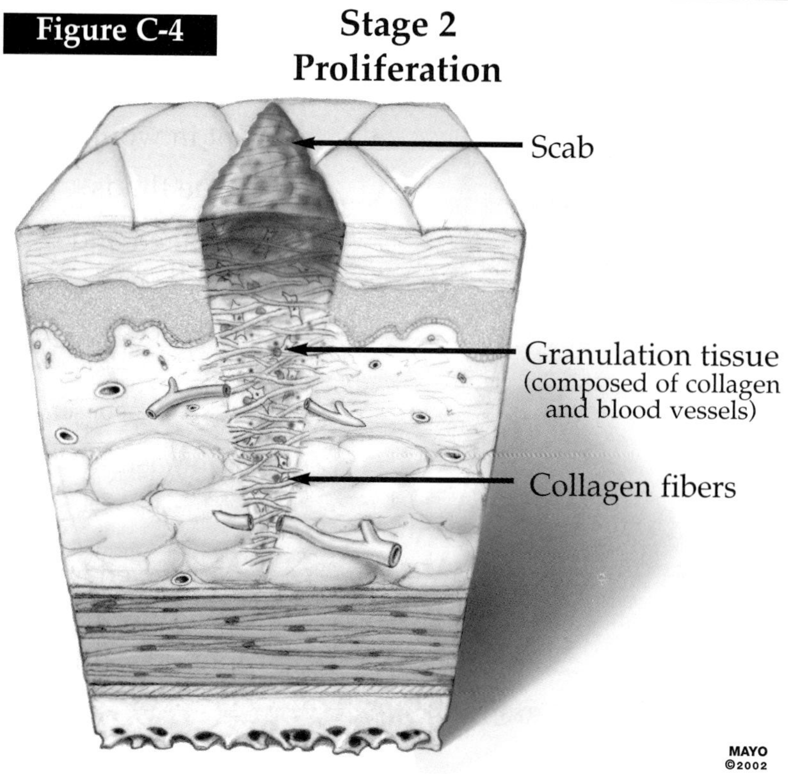

c. Stage 3, Scar Maturation (day 21 to 1 year)
The fibroblasts produce collagen. Collagen constitutes the major substance of connective tissue, and it is the collagen that needs to remodel across the wounded tissues to increase the tensile strength of the wound. It's the collagen scar (**cicatrix**) that determines the final strength of the wound **(Figure C-5)**.

A summary of the 3 stages of wound healing is seen in **Figure C-6**.

2. Wound Classification

Wounds are classified according to the estimate of bacterial contamination and the possible risk of infection. Wound classification includes four types of wounds.

a. Clean wounds
Most wounds created in surgery are made in a sterile environment and are rarely infected. Incision and wound closure using sutures is termed **"closure by primary intention."** Primary intention is the method of choice for closing a wound. This type of closure carries minimal risk of postoperative complications, since the surgery is performed under sterile conditions.

b. Clean contaminated wounds
If during the course of an operation a muccus membrane lined cavity is entered, you have a clean wound that is now contaminated. For example, if the oral pharyngeal cavity (upper aerodigestive tract), genitourinary (GU), or gastrointestinal (GI) tract is entered, then you have a wound that was initially clean but is now contaminated by virtue of entry into a field contaminated with bacteria. A common operation, appendectomy, is an example of a clean contaminated wound.

Figure C-4

**Stage 2
Proliferation**

Scab

Granulation tissue
(composed of collagen
and blood vessels)

Collagen fibers

MAYO
©2002

14

C. The Wound

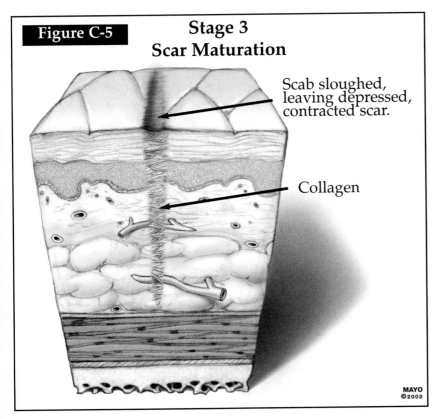

Figure C-5

Stage 3
Scar Maturation

Scab sloughed, leaving depressed, contracted scar.

Collagen

MAYO
©2002

c. Contaminated wounds

Contaminated wounds are wounds in which there is **already** exposure to microorganisms. Examples of contaminated wounds are traumatic injuries, open fractures, or entry into the genitourinary tract (GU), the gastrointestinal (GI) tract, or **biliary** tract. These contaminated wounds may become infected.

d. Infected wounds

Infected wounds are also called "dirty" wounds because they are already growing bacteria, and pus has developed. They are clinically infected before surgery is performed. For example, an abscess is an infected wound. Wounds with **devitalized** or dying tissue are also already infected. Infection at the time of operation can increase the postoperative complication rate considerably.

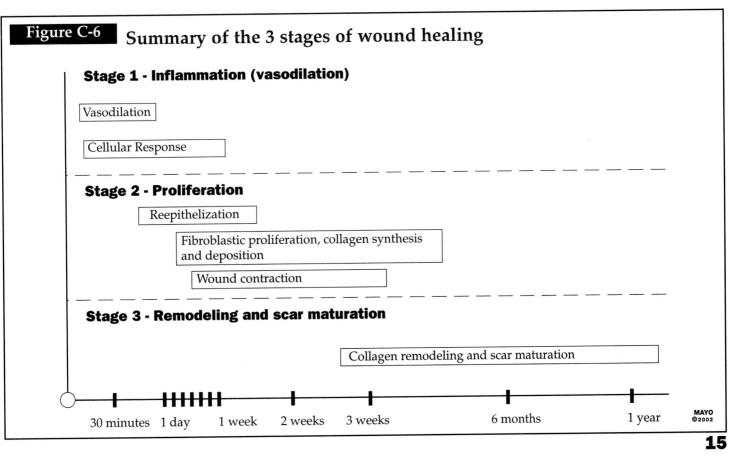

Figure C-6 Summary of the 3 stages of wound healing

Stage 1 - Inflammation (vasodilation)

Vasodilation

Cellular Response

Stage 2 - Proliferation

Reepithelization

Fibroblastic proliferation, collagen synthesis and deposition

Wound contraction

Stage 3 - Remodeling and scar maturation

Collagen remodeling and scar maturation

30 minutes | 1 day | 1 week | 2 weeks | 3 weeks | 6 months | 1 year

MAYO
©2002

C. The Wound

3. Factors That Affect Wound Healing

There is a need to know those factors which are basic to all operative procedures that may affect both the results of the surgery and well-being of the patient.

a. Age
The patient's age may affect wound healing. Children tend to heal with a robust response and may get **hypertrophic scars**. As the years pass, metabolic changes occur that are associated with both vascular insufficiencies and a lack of tissue elasticity. Because of these factors, old age may prolong or delay the healing of a wound.

b. Weight
Excessive fat may prevent adequate wound closure. Fat itself has a reduced blood supply and, therefore, makes the patient vulnerable to infection and/or a delay in healing.

c. Nutrition
Proteins, vitamins, and adequate hydration are all necessary to promote wound healing. Deficiencies in any of these important elements may disturb and delay wound healing.

d. Dehydration
Adequate **electrolyte** balance and fluid levels are crucial to both kidney and cardiac function. The basic **metabolic** processes of the body require proper fluid balance to promote wound healing.

e. Blood supply
Adequate blood supply to the wound site is necessary to promote wound healing. Poor circulation, diabetes, or other vascular illnesses may diminish the blood supply to the wound and can result in a delay in healing.

f. Immune responses
Immune response deficiencies may signifi-cantly compromise surgical procedures. Patients who have **HIV**, who have been on high dosages of steroids for a prolonged period of time or who have had chemotherapy may have a deficient immune response. These factors may interfere with and delay the healing process.

g. Chronic illness
Patients who have concomitant systemic illness or **endocrine** disorders such as diabetes are more likely to have postoperative complications with prolonged or delayed healing. Other situations involving systemic illness, including malignancies, may complicate wound healing.

h. Drugs and radiation therapy
Steroids, immunosuppressive drugs, **antineoplastic** drugs, or **radiation therapy** may significantly disturb and delay wound healing.

i. Smoking
Smoking can cause lung complications and it can prolong and disturb wound healing. Patients who do smoke should stop one week before surgery to prevent complications. Ideally smoking should be totally terminated.

4. Healing

Fundamentally there are three types or methods of healing. (See **Figure C-7,** summary of the 3 methods of wound healing.)

a. Primary intention
As mentioned, healing by primary intention is that which follows surgical wound closure with sutures. Uncomplicated healing by primary intention occurs with minimal edema, minimal discharge, and no bacterial infection. The tensile strength of the wound increases significantly, and the skin obtains approximately 80% of its tensile strength before the wounding. Healing by primary intention is the most desirable to the surgeon.

C. The Wound

Figure C-7

SUMMARY OF THREE METHODS OF HEALING

a. HEALING BY PRIMARY INTENTION

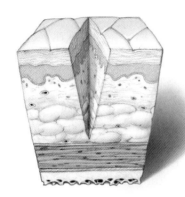 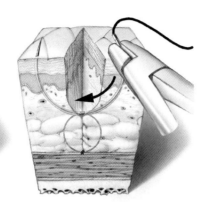 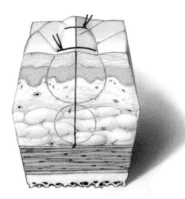

Surgical wound (knife)	Suturing	Surgical closure (immediate)

b. HEALING BY SECONDARY INTENTION

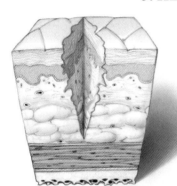 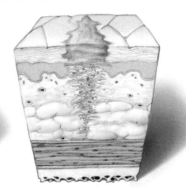 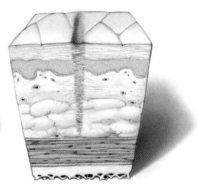

Rough wound (injury)	Granulation tissue closes wound without sutures	No surgical closure, depressed scar formation

c. HEALING BY TERTIARY INTENTION

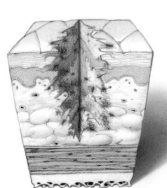 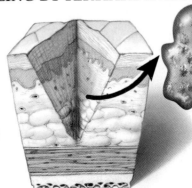 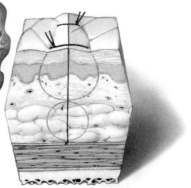

Rough wound (deep injury)	Surgical debridement (delayed 4-6 days post injury)	Surgical closure (delayed)

MAYO
©2002

17

C. The Wound

b. Secondary intention

If the healing does not occur by primary intention and the wound is left to granulate closed, this is termed healing by secondary intention. Healing by secondary intention occurs when the wound is left open and the healing proceeds with **granulation tissue** from the deeper layers out toward the surface of the skin. Healing by secondary intention is a slower process and usually takes four to eight weeks to re-epithelialize the area.

c. Tertiary intention

This is also termed **delayed primary closure**. This is the method of choice in contaminated, dirty, infected wounds with loss of tissue. The surgeon may debride the nonviable tissue before closure. Surgical closure with sutures is usually performed about four to six days after injury. Unlike secondary intention, the wound is closed with delayed suturing, rather than being allowed to close entirely by granulation.

d. Complications

Significant problems that complicate healing are: infection, wound breakdown (**dehiscence**), **hematoma**, **seroma**, **hypertrophic scars** and **keloids**. Organisms that find their way into the wound may produce delayed healing, generalized **bacteremia**, **gangrene**, or even death. Antibiotics alone may be used when **cellulitis** occurs. If abscess or **necrosis** occurs, the wound must first be incised and drained with removal (**debridement**) of dead tissue before healing can occur. Wound **dehiscence** may occur in areas prone to movement, in elderly patients, in the debilitated patients, or can result from inappropriate or improper suture techniques.

A **hematoma** is a collection of blood in the depths of a wound, while a seroma is a collection of serous fluid in the depths of a wound. Hematomas usually result from inadequate **hemostasis** at surgery, or reopening of a blood vessel after surgery. Some factors predisposing to hematoma formation include hypertension (high blood pressure), bleeding disorders and presence of excessive dead space in a wound. Untreated, hematomas may lead to abscess formation, loss of skin (**slough**), or excessive scar tissue. When recognized, hematomas **must** be treated expeditiously by reopening and draining the blood out of the wound.

Seroma is a collection of **serum** in the tissues. This usually occurs in the normal wound healing process. The risk of excessive seroma formation can be decreased by careful closure of all of the layers of the wound and by immobilizing the wound during the healing phase. Close all dead spaces. If they occur, seromas should also be drained to prevent infection and further complications. Sometimes this can be done with a needle and syringe, while other times the wound must be reopened.

Hypertrophic scars and **keloids** are erythematous, tender, elevated, unsightly scars that may itch or produce a contraction cicatrix. The clinical difference between the two is that a keloid extends beyond the margins of the initial scar while a hypertrophic scar does not. Many treatments are available for each and include surgical scar revision, pressure dressings, and steroid injections. Further discussion of these entities is beyond the scope of this work.

Quiz

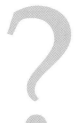

Fill in the shaded blanks! See page 10, Figure B-1 for the correct answers.

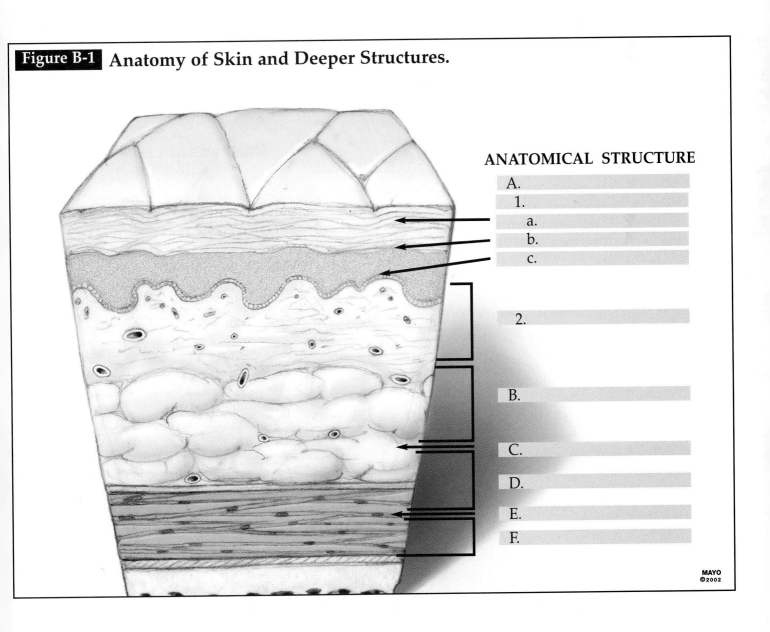

Figure B-1 Anatomy of Skin and Deeper Structures.

ANATOMICAL STRUCTURE

A.

  1.

    a.

    b.

    c.

  2.

B.

C.

D.

E.

F.

MAYO
©2002

D. Basic Principles in Surgery

There are a number of basic surgical principles that you must be aware of when performing surgery.

1. Hemostasis

Bleeding is the enemy of proper visualization (exposure) during surgery. If you can't see, you can't operate safely. A "dry" (bloodless) surgical field is crucial for adequate visualization. In addition, when the surgical field is dry, the accumulation of serum or blood is minimal. If blood does accumulate in the wound after the surgical procedure it can become a hematoma. Hematoma can lead to infection or to a delay in wound healing. It **must** be drained.

2. Handling of the Tissues

Be gentle to the tissues! Use a dissection technique that produces minimal tissue trauma. It is also crucial to preserve all vital structures including nerves, blood vessels (arteries and veins), connective tissue, and muscles. Retraction (pulling on the tissues) should be firm yet gentle since injury to tissues can impair wound healing and allow bacteria to colonize.

3. Incision Planning

Why do we incise the skin? Actually, surgeons make incisions for a variety of reasons. The reasons include excision (surgical removal) of skin lesions, exposure of deeper structures for other surgical procedures, and reconstruction of traumatic defects. Yet, prior to making any incision, planning is necessary. As the surgeon, you must choose an incision that will accomplish several goals. First, the incision chosen must result in the best scar. The best scar is the least noticeable and has the least interference with function. A well-planned incision will allow you to adequately expose the underlying structures and avoid injury to critical deeper structures like major nerves, arteries, veins, and vital organs.

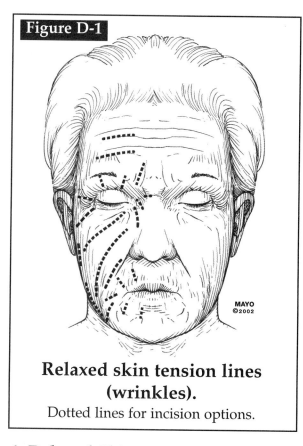

Figure D-1

Relaxed skin tension lines (wrinkles).
Dotted lines for incision options.

4. Relaxed Skin Tension Lines

A good scar results when the skin incisions are made along the lines (axis) of the relaxed skin tension lines (**Figure D-1, D-2**). Relaxed skin tension lines are the lines of minimal tension of the skin. Incisions should be made on or parallel to these lines so that they are under the least possible tension while healing and produce a minimal scar. The technique used in the incision itself and the amount of wound closing tension are also critical things to consider in order to produce a minimal or less noticeable scar. As far as the incision itself, it needs to be planned well before a knife is utilized — thus the dictum **"decision before incision."**

Incisions parallel to relaxed skin tension lines, along **aesthetic unit boundaries** and in the midline of the face and body heal with less perceptible scarring. The aesthetic boundaries or aesthetic units of the face include things like the cheek and the lip

D. Basic Principles in Surgery

Figure D-2 Relaxed skin tension lines —
Lines for incision placement.

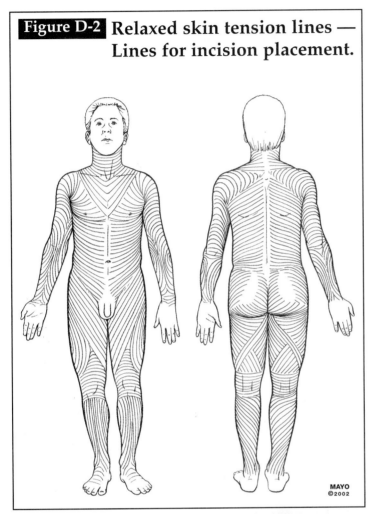

MAYO
©2002

boundary (the nasolabial groove) and the border of the eyebrow where there are natural shadows and contour changes to help camouflage or hide a scar **(Figure D-3)**.

The nose is a "unit" by itself and is subdivided further into smaller surfaces or subunits including: 1) sidewalls 2)dorsum 3) tip and 4) alae **(Figure D-3)**.

As far as the incision itself is concerned, the scalpel should be used to make a skin cut perpendicular to the skin edge and not slanted or **beveled**. In rare circumstances, the surgeon intentionally bevels the skin edge. A beveled edge is usually more difficult to close surgically with good apposition of the wound edges close together. The incision perpendicular to the skin edge is easier to get good apposition of the wound edges which results in a better (less noticeable) scar.

5. Undermining

After incision or excision, undermining (relaxing or loosening) of the skin edges surrounding the defect assists in wound closure **(Figure D-4, 1-7)**. This is because the wound edges can be brought together under less stress or tension by combining both deep (subcutaneous or subcuticular) sutures and skin sutures. Also, the act of undermining itself relaxes the skin so that it is under less tension.

Figure D-3

Aesthetic Unit Boundaries of the Face

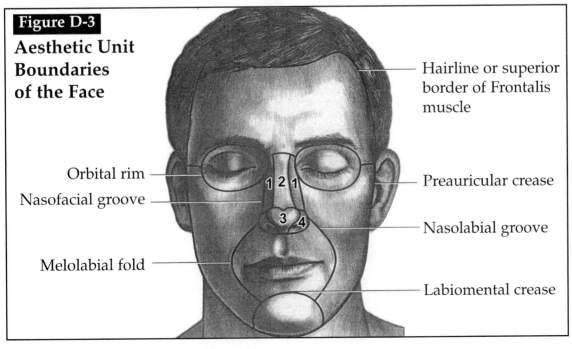

Orbital rim

Nasofacial groove

Melolabial fold

Hairline or superior border of Frontalis muscle

Preauricular crease

Nasolabial groove

Labiomental crease

21

D. Basic Principles in Surgery

Figure D-4

1

Undermine with scissors

1 - 2 cm

Undermining below skin

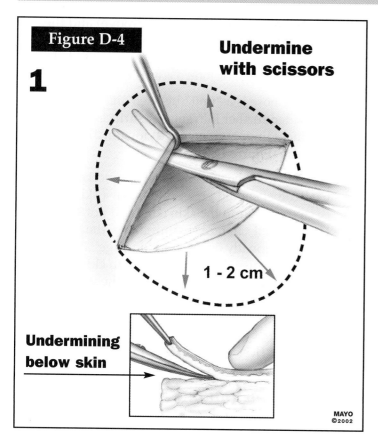

MAYO
©2002

Figure D-4

2

Undermined

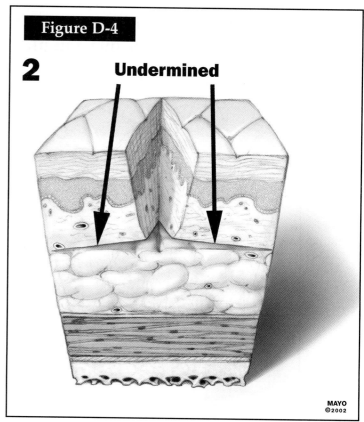

MAYO
©2002

Figure D-4

3

Deep closure

Cut edge

Cut edge

Needle enters far from cut edge

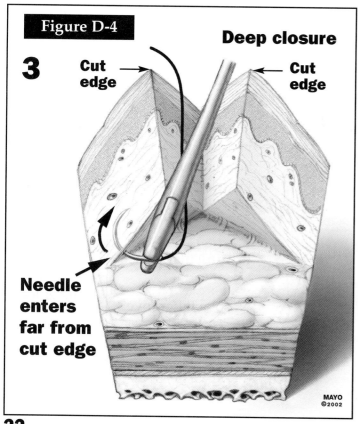

MAYO
©2002

Figure D-4

4

Needle exits near edge

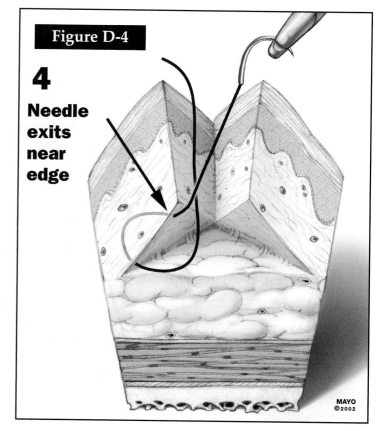

MAYO
©2002

D. Basic Principles in Surgery

Figure D-4

5

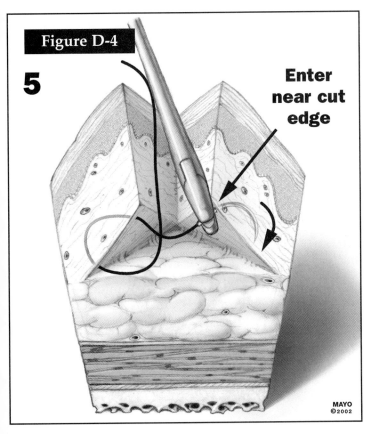

Enter near cut edge

MAYO
©2002

Figure D-4

6

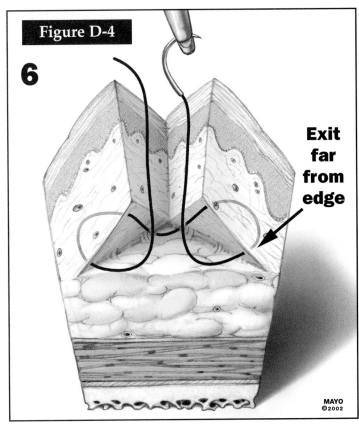

Exit far from edge

MAYO
©2002

Figure D-4

7

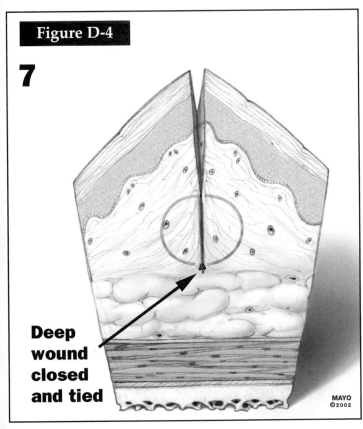

Deep wound closed and tied

MAYO
©2002

23

D. Basic Principles in Surgery

6. Choice of Suture Materials

The proper suture material is required so that the tissues in each layer can be adequately brought together, also termed in apposition or approximated (*See SECTION H, Sutures, Needles and Knots pgs. 55-120*). Suture materials maximize healing by approximating (bringing together) the tissues being operated on. The reaction of the body to various suture materials may be either minimal or intense. Intense tissue reaction involves swelling (edema) that can delay healing. Careful and precise suture placement, with the proper amount of tension, promotes healing with minimal scar tissue formation.

7. Closing With Sufficient Tension

It is important to approximate the wound, which means to bring the edges of the wound in close proximity to each other, but not too tightly. The dictum **"approximate, don't strangulate"** guides the surgeon during closure. You will learn the feel of the proper amount of tension required to close a wound. Excessive tissue tension or tissue strangulation can also be uncomfortable to the patient and may lead to infection and delayed healing.

8. Tissue Moisture

Long (many hours) procedures may require periodic lavage (washing) of the operative field with warm saline to maintain moisture and prevent drying of tissue.

9. Debriding Necrotic (Dead) Tissue

All **devitalized** (necrotic) tissue needs to be removed so that healing can occur, especially in traumatized wounds. For example, foreign bodies, including road debris, dirt, glass, and wood fragments, need to be debrided (removed) before you close the wound so the possibility of infection is markedly reduced.

D. Basic Principles in Surgery

10. Dead Spaces

Dead spaces are areas in the wound that have not been adequately closed. It is important that each layer be closed individually, especially in the fatty layers. Dead space facilitates wound separation, seroma or hematoma formation, and bacterial overgrowth **(Figure D-5)**. It may be necessary to either apply a pressure dressing or insert a drain (or both) to help eliminate dead space even after adequate closure of the tissues has been performed.

11. Postoperative Wound Stress

Postoperative activity can produce excessive tension on the wound during the healing phase. Therefore, it is sometimes necessary to immobilize the wound to prevent suture breakdown and **dehiscence** (breakdown) of the wound. Wound breakdown can occur if the patient coughs or strains postoperatively. Immobilization of the wound can facilitate healing and minimize scar formation.

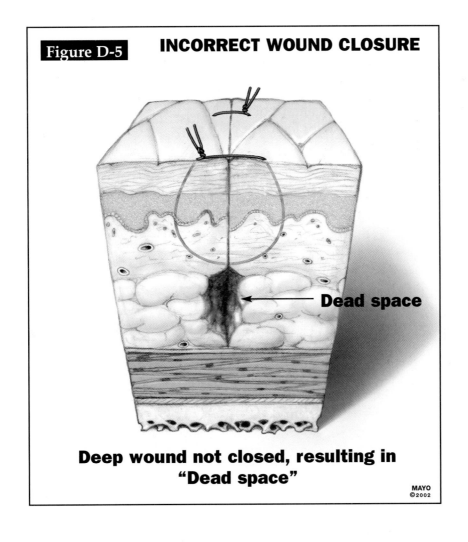

Figure D-5 INCORRECT WOUND CLOSURE

← Dead space

Deep wound not closed, resulting in "Dead space"

MAYO
©2002

E. Local Anesthetics

1. Anesthetics

Local anesthetics are used extensively in surgery. When used in combination with **vasoconstrictive** agents they may reduce surgical blood loss. They can also reduce **perioperative** and **postoperative** pain, reduce nausea and vomiting associated with general anesthetics, reduce **cardiopulmonary** risk, and allow earlier discharge from the hospital. Patients who are good candidates for local anesthetics are people who can cooperate with the surgeon and calmly follow directions. Patients who are **not** good candidates for local anesthetics include children, anxious adults, severely emotionally disturbed patients, and patients with a language barrier. These individuals should probably have surgery done under general anesthesia.

The mechanism of action of local anesthetic agents is to block nerve conduction. This prevents the sensation of pain. Local anesthetics can be used by infiltration (injection) through various sizes (gauges) and lengths of needles **(Table E-1, Figures E-1 and E-2)**. **Table E-2 and E-3** list the common local anesthetic drugs used for infiltration or for topical application.

Table E-1

CHART OF COMMON NEEDLE SIZES

Gauge refers to the diameter of the needle bore. The smaller the number, the bigger the diameter. Therefore, a 15-gauge needle is a larger bore diameter than a 27-gauge needle. The length of the needle ranges from 1/4" to spinal needles of about 3". **See Figures E-1 and E-2.**

Example of the bore diameter of 18-gauge needle ●

Example of the bore diameter of 20-gauge needle ●

Example of the bore diameter of 22-gauge needle ●

Example of the bore diameter of 24-gauge needle •

Example of the bore diameter of 26-gauge needle •

Example of the bore diameter of 30-gauge needle •

(note: not exact sizes)

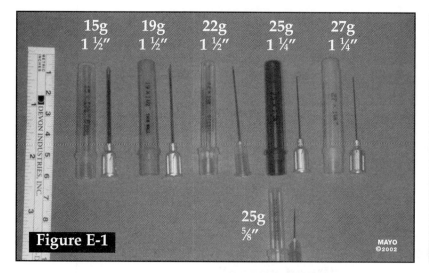

Figure E-1

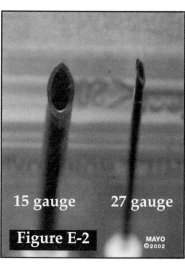

Figure E-2

Note: various needle lengths and gauge sizes (diameter of bore)

E. Local Anesthetics

Table E-2

Local Anesthetic Drugs for <u>INFILTRATION</u>

	Maximum dose* without epinephrine by body weight, mg/kg	Onset	Approximate duration	Average adult dose, mg
Lidocaine (Xylocaine®)	4.5 mg/kg	Immediate	2 hours	500
Bupivacaine (Marcaine®)	3 mg/kg	2 to 5 min	4 hours	100
Procaine (Novocaine®)	15 mg/kg	2 to 5 min	1 hour	1000

*Maximum dosage limits must be individualized in each patient. **Epinephrine** is a **vasoconstrictive** agent that allows an increased amount of local anesthesia to be injected.

Example: To calculate the maximum dose of lidocaine the weight of the person must be known.

For a 70-kg person (154 lb) the maximum dose of lidocaine, with epinephrine is 7 mg/kg (4.5 mg/kg without epinephrine). Therefore, 7 mg x 70 kg = 490 mg for a 70-kg person.

1% solution = 10 mg/cc**, so 30 cc of 1% lidocaine is safe because 30 cc of 1% lidocaine is 300 mg of lidocaine, which is less than the maximum dose, 490 mg.

---

*WARNING: This table in no way implies that these dosages are safe or absolute maximums. Systemic reactions can be encountered with much smaller doses, but much larger doses, used judiciously, have been administered without ill effects.

Adapted from Moore DC, Bridenbaugh LD, Thompson GE, et al: Factors determining dosages of amide-type local anesthetic drugs. Anesthesiology 1977; 47:263-268; in de Jong RH: Local Anesthetics, p 353. St. Louis, Mosby-Year Book, 1994.

From Brown DL: Regional Anesthesia and Analgesia. p. 140, Section II, Basic Sciences of Regional Anesthetics. W.B. Saunders Co., 1996.

** "Kern's Rule"
Percent of drug x 10 = mg of drug per cc

Example: *Question*: How many milligrams of lidocaine are there in a 2% lidocaine solution?

Answer: A 2% lidocaine solution = 20 mg of lidocaine per cc.

MAYO
©2002

E. Local Anesthetics

Table E-3

Local Anesthetic Drugs for <u>TOPICAL</u> <u>APPLICATION</u>

For MUCOSA   **Maximum dose***

    Lidocaine (Xylocaine®)   200 mg (5 cc of a 4% solution)

    Cocaine   200 mg (4 cc of a 5% solution or 2 cc of a 10% solution)

    Tetracaine   100 mg (5 cc of a 2% solution)

For SKIN --- Local Anesthetic Drugs for Topical Use on Skin

    EMLA Cream (lidocaine 2.5% plus prilocaine 2.5%)

    Apply 1 hour before needle insertion. Duration is 1-2 hours.

    Maximum recommended application area is based on body weight:

Body weight (kg)	Maximum application area, cm^2
Up to 10 kg	100
10 - 20 kg	600
Above 20 kg	2000

***WARNING:** This table in no way implies that these dosages are safe or absolute maximums. Systemic reactions can be encountered with much smaller doses, but much larger doses, used judiciously, have been administered without ill effects.

E. Local Anesthetics

2. Injection technique

There is a method of drawing up the local anesthetic into your syringe. Select a large bore needle (example 18 gauge) to draw the anesthetic solution into your syringe **(Figure E-3)**. First inject about 3 cc of air into the bottle **(Figure E-4)**. Then pull back the plunger of the syringe to draw the anesthetic fluid (solution) into the syringe **(Figure E-5)**. Usually about 5 cc of anesthetic solution is a good start for most procedures.

When inserting local anesthetics it is reasonable to give a **test dose** to make sure no adverse reactions occur. Use the smallest needle size possible to minimize the discomfort. Clean the skin with an alcohol preparation. Penetrate the skin, and advance the needle slowly. Inject and **then** advance so you push the anesthetic into the tissues and **then** advance the needle **(Figure E-6)**. Be sure to discard the needle in a **sharps container** to prevent accidents. This technique is almost painless when using a 27 g or 30 g (smallest) needle and injecting slowly.

If too much local anesthetic agent is used, toxicity can occur. The signs and symptoms of toxicity must be known by every person who gives these agents. These issues are very important but are beyond the scope of this text.

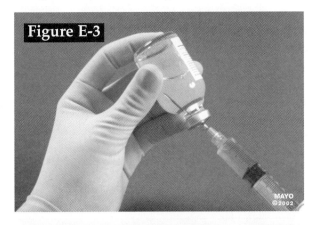

Figure E-3

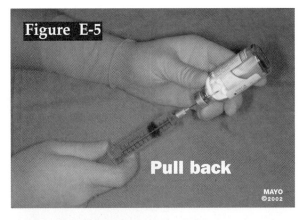

Figure E-5

Pull back

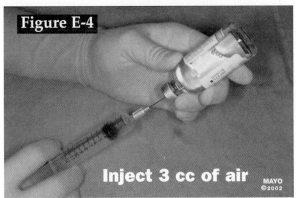

Figure E-4

Inject 3 cc of air

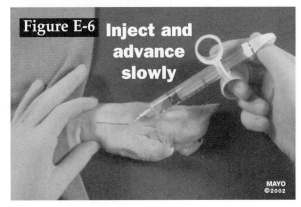

Figure E-6 Inject and advance slowly

F. Scrubbing

1. Washing Your Hands

Prior to scrubbing, always place the surgical scrub suit cap of your choice on your head. All your hair should be covered. Eye protection is required. Be sure to defog your lenses and secure a piece of tape partially over the skin on your nose and partially over your surgical mask to hold the mask in place and minimize fogging of the lenses. Despite different mask styles, they all have a horizontal metal bar that you can tighten over your nose **(Figure F-1,2)** to prevent fogging. Now find the scrub sink **(Figure F-3).**

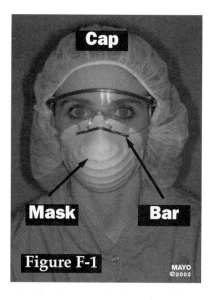

Cap
Mask   Bar
Figure F-1   MAYO ©2002

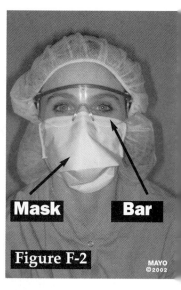

Mask   Bar
Figure F-2   MAYO ©2002

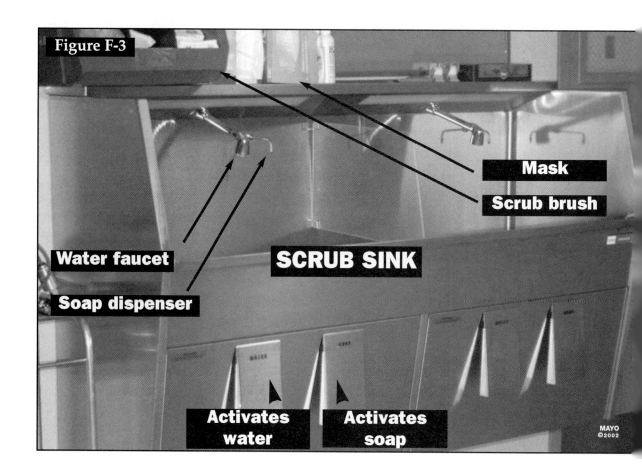

Figure F-3

Mask
Scrub brush
Water faucet   SCRUB SINK
Soap dispenser
Activates water   Activates soap   MAYO ©2002

F. Scrubbing

The soap, brush and sponge combination are frequently prepackaged. Open the package **(Figures F-4-6)**. The water is turned on by either an automatic switch or a foot or leg switch **(Figure F-7)**. A nail cleaner is typically enclosed in the package. The fingernails are cleaned. Both forearms are wetted up to the elbows, and the foam is formed on the brush **(Figures F-8-11)**.

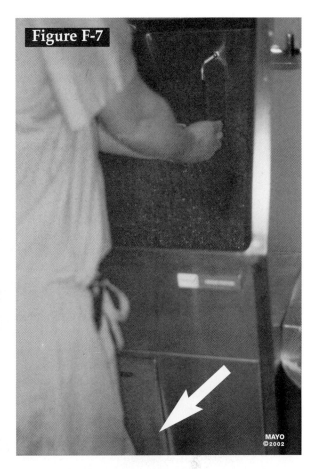

Knee activates water flow and turns it off.

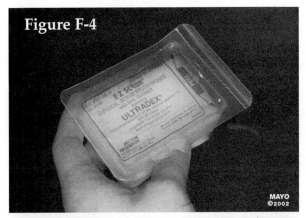

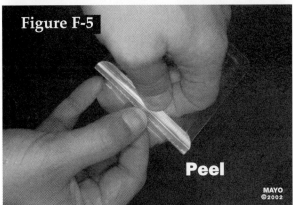

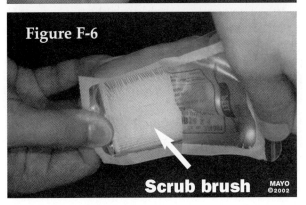

F. Scrubbing

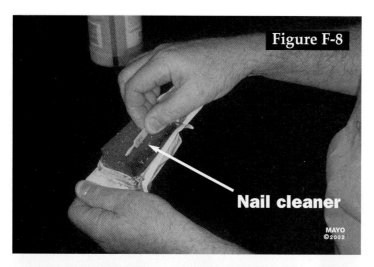

Figure F-8

Nail cleaner

MAYO
©2002

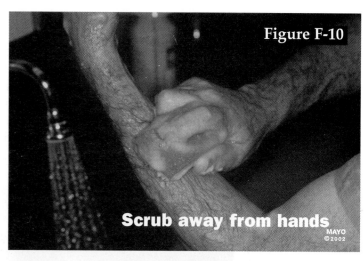

Figure F-10

Scrub away from hands

MAYO
©2002

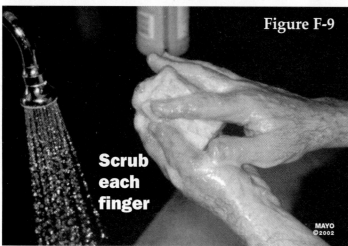

Figure F-9

Scrub
each
finger

MAYO
©2002

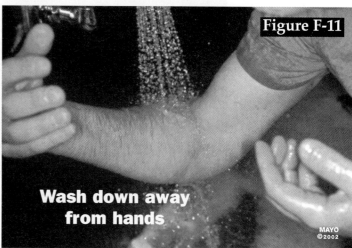

Figure F-11

Wash down away
from hands

MAYO
©2002

After the fingernails are cleansed, the sponge is used to scrub each finger 10 times on each side of each finger on each hand (**Figure F-9**). The scrub is then carried further up the hands and forearms (**Figure F-10**). The scrub is carried up to the level of the elbow. The other hand is then done in the same fashion with care to clean all sides of the fingers, between the fingers, the hands, wrists, forearms, and up to the elbows. The sponge is discarded, and the hands are first raised, then rinsed.

You can bend over to rinse the arms while holding your hands upright so that the water runs towards the elbow, **not** back down toward the hand. Why not? The hands are held upright to prevent the soap and water adjacent to the unscrubbed, unsterile elbow region from running back and contaminating the hands (**Figure F-11**).

One arm is then dried from the fingers and hands **toward** the forearm and elbow. The towel is then turned and grasped in the clean area. The same drying procedure is carried out on the opposite arm and hand. Care is taken **NEVER** to dry back from the unsterile elbow region toward the clean hands.

F. Scrubbing

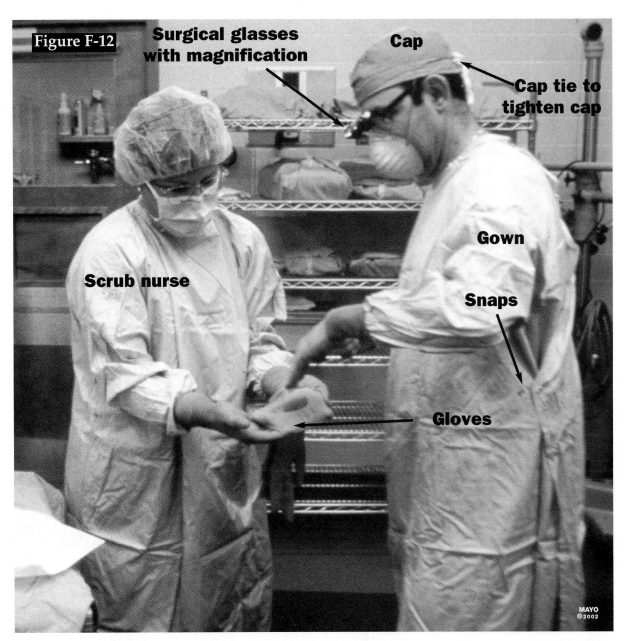

Figure F-12

Surgical glasses with magnification

Cap

Cap tie to tighten cap

Gown

Snaps

Scrub nurse

Gloves

MAYO
©2002

 ## 2. Gowning

The scrub nurse holds up the gown and the surgeon inserts his/her arms. The sterile assistant pulls the gown sleeves so that the surgeon's hands become exposed.

 ## 3. Gloving

Gloves come in various sizes. The most common sizes range from the smaller 6 1/2 to the larger 8. Try a few sizes to see which is best for you. After the gown is put on, the gloves are held open by the scrub nurse for sterile entry (Figure F-12). Utilizing the first gloved hand, the surgeon can assist the placement of the second glove. A circulating nurse then snaps up the gown for the surgeon. The sterile ties around the gown or snaps can be fixed either by the surgeon or by the scrub nurse to preserve sterility.

G. Surgical Instruments

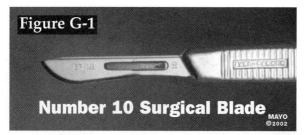

Figure G-1

Number 10 Surgical Blade
MAYO
©2002

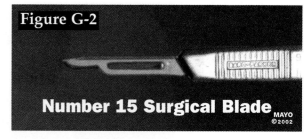

Figure G-2

Number 15 Surgical Blade
MAYO
©2002

1. Scalpel

The scalpel is the instrument most synonymous with the surgeon. It is composed of a scalpel blade and a handle. Scalpels are used to make incisions in the skin or other deeper structures when a fine and precise cut is required. Scalpel blades can also be used to dissect (separate) various types of tissue.

Scalpel blades come in multiple shapes and sizes. The two most common blades are the #10 **(Figure G-1)** and the #15 **(Figure G-2)**.

The Number 10 blade is a large knife blade used for incisions on the scalp and body. The belly of the blade is the cutting edge. The scalpel handle is held like a steak knife **(Figure G-3)**: the index finger guides the blade while the handle is held between the middle finger and thumb in the palm of the hand.

The Number 15 blade is a smaller knife blade. It is typically used for facial surgery. This blade is held like a pencil **(Figure G-4)**. An incision is started by inserting the blade into the skin like a stab. Then the knife handle is rotated backwards so the cutting belly of the blade is held at approximately a 45-degree angle to the skin surface during the incision.

How do you load a scalpel blade onto a scalpel handle? Answer: Grasp the blade with a hemostat clamp near the base of the sharp cutting edge of the blade **(Figure G-5)**. Then advance the blade onto the scalpel handle **(Figure G-5)**. To unload the scalpel blade, grasp the blade with the hemostat clamp **(Figure G-6)**, then rotate the hemostat clamp to lift the blade and advance (push) forward and remove the blade **(Figure G-6)**.

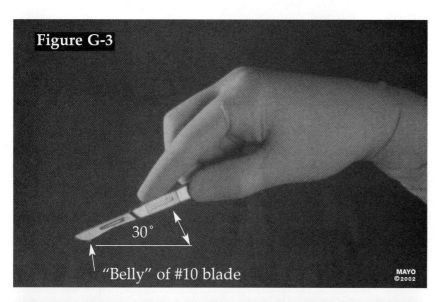

Figure G-3

30°

"Belly" of #10 blade

MAYO
©2002

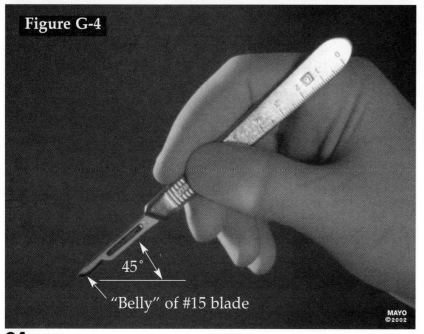

Figure G-4

45°

"Belly" of #15 blade

MAYO
©2002

G. Surgical Instruments

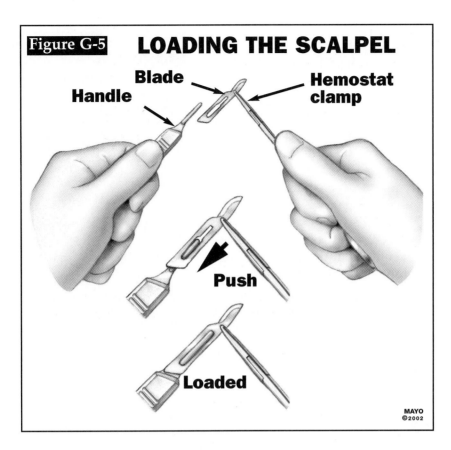

Figure G-5 — **LOADING THE SCALPEL**

Handle

Blade

Hemostat clamp

Push

Loaded

MAYO
©2002

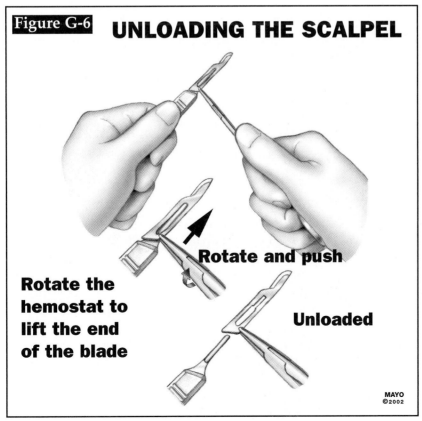

Figure G-6 — **UNLOADING THE SCALPEL**

Rotate and push

Rotate the hemostat to lift the end of the blade

Unloaded

MAYO
©2002

G. Surgical Instruments

2. *Tissue Scissors*

Tissue scissors (also called dissection scissors or undermining scissors) are used to separate (dissect) the tissues. This elevation or separation of the tissues is called undermining. Many tissue scissors are curved at the cutting edge **(Figures G-7-9)**. If they are curved at the cutting edge, it is best to dissect and undermine with the curved tips **upward** so you can visualize exactly what is being cut. Dissection scissors usually have tips that are either partially blunted or fully blunted to prevent penetration of structures beyond the surgeon's view **(Figures G-8, 9)**. When dissecting with tissue scissors, appropriate tension and countertension on the wound edges are necessary for precise undermining.

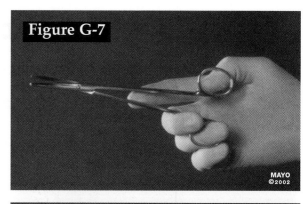

Figure G-7

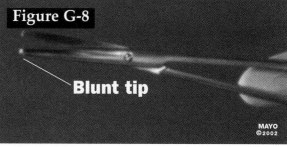

Figure G-8

Blunt tip

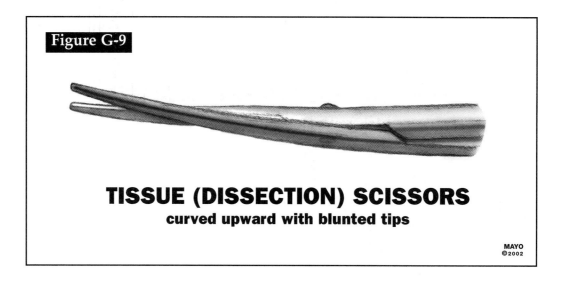

Figure G-9

TISSUE (DISSECTION) SCISSORS
curved upward with blunted tips

G. Surgical Instruments

3. Forceps

The forceps is used to grasp, retract, or stabilize tissue. The forceps is gripped between the thumb and middle finger while the index finger is utilized for stabilization **(Figure G-10)**. Various types of forceps are available. They come either with no teeth, single tooth, or multiple teeth on the end of the instrument **(Figure G-11)**. Various tooth sizes are used depending on the size and nature of the tissues to be handled. When grasping tissue, choose a forceps with a tooth size appropriate for the delicacy of the tissue to be handled **(Figure G-11)**. If possible, when operating on skin, use forceps to grasp the dermis (tissue just below the surface) rather than the epidermis (the skin surface itself). This grasping of the dermis helps to prevent marking and injuring the skin at the wound edge with the forceps.

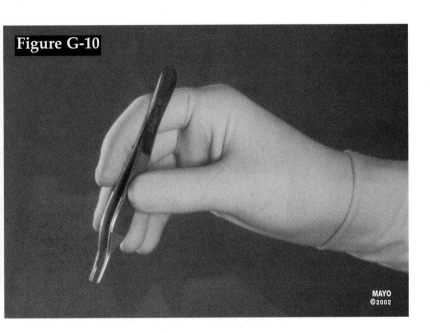

Figure G-10

MAYO
©2002

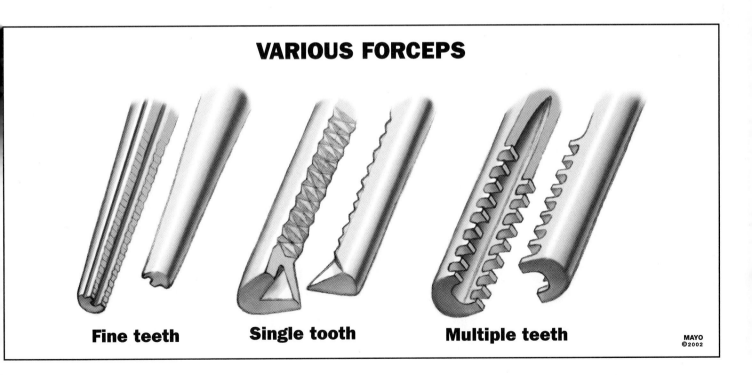

VARIOUS FORCEPS

Fine teeth   **Single tooth**   **Multiple teeth**

MAYO
©2002

G. Surgical Instruments

4. Skin Hooks

Skin hooks are sharp instruments used for pulling (also called retracting) tissues **(Figure G-12)**. Retracting allows you to see the deeper tissues, and also puts the tissues on tension, which can help in the surgical dissection with a knife or tissue scissors. Most skin hooks have small, sharp prongs that hook into the dermis. This prevents trauma to the epidermis during wound retraction.

The hooks are placed and retraction is performed by grasping the instrument between the thumb and index finger. The middle finger can stabilize the hook **(Figure G-13)** or can be used to place countertraction on the tissue beyond the skin hook for better visibility and easier dissection. Some examples of the various skin hooks are noted **(Figure G-14)**.

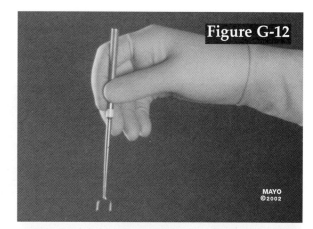

Figure G-12

MAYO
©2002

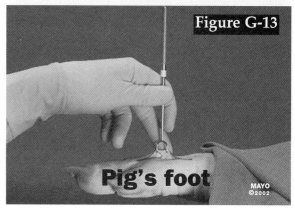

Figure G-13

Pig's foot

MAYO
©2002

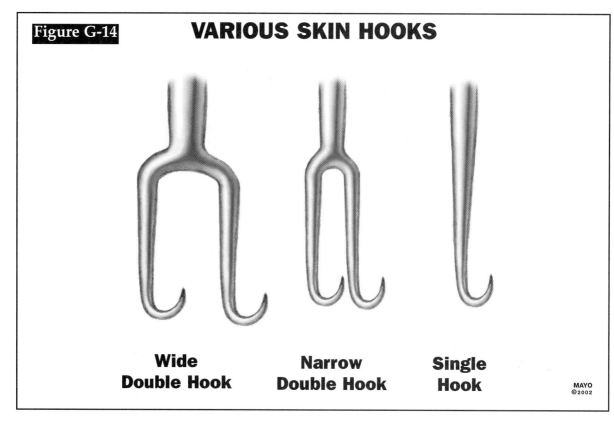

Figure G-14   **VARIOUS SKIN HOOKS**

Wide Double Hook   **Narrow Double Hook**   **Single Hook**

MAYO
©2002

G. Surgical Instruments

5. Retractor

The retractor is a blunt instrument used to pull tissues out of the way **(Figure G-15)**. They come in all shapes and sizes and some are even self-retaining.

Pulling the tissue in one direction is called **traction**. Pulling the tissue in opposite directions is called **counter-traction**. Both traction and counter-traction can be accomplished with either an instrument or finger (pulling with tension) **(Figure G-16)**. Traction and counter traction facilitates dissection of tissue.

Figure G-15

MAYO
©2002

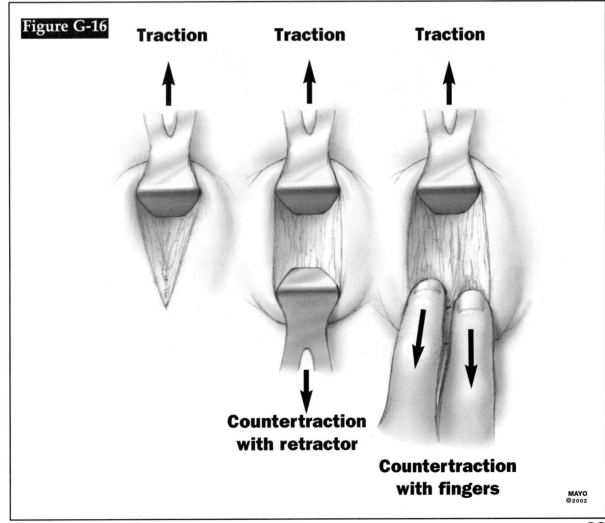

Figure G-16

Traction   Traction   Traction

Countertraction
with retractor

Countertraction
with fingers

MAYO
©2002

G. Surgical Instruments

6. Needle Holder (Needle Driver)

The needle holder is the instrument used for placing sutures. Actually, the needle holder, also called a needle driver, holds the needle and pushes or drives the needle with the attached suture through the tissues.

The needle holder is held in the palm with the thumb and fourth finger in the rings (holes) of the handle **(Figure G-17)**. The second finger is utilized to stabilize the direction of the needle holder's end. The third finger is placed against the ring, with the fourth finger used to stabilize the holding of the needle holder.

The needle with the suture attached is usually grasped in the jaws of the needle holder at about two-thirds from the pointed tip of the needle **(Figure G-18)**. This allows stabilization of the needle and helps prevent bending of the needle.

Needle holders may have several varieties of jaws **(Figure G-19)**. The first are jaws with teeth for stability. The second has particles such as tungsten carbide for needle stability to prevent rotation or slipping of the needle in the jaws. Third are smooth jaws (without teeth). A smooth, fine-jawed needle holder is used with fine needles, and a heavier, wider-jawed needle holder with teeth is selected for a heavier needle. The needle holder can also be used to tie and knot sutures. **Do not** use a hemostat as a needle holder. Hemostat jaws are not designed to hold a needle and may **damage** the needle.

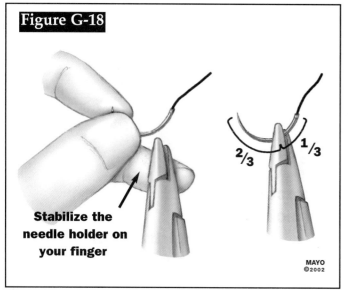

Figure G-17

Stabilize the needle holder with index (second) finger

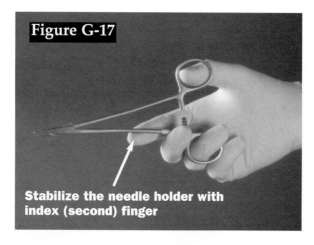

Figure G-18

Stabilize the needle holder on your finger

2/3 1/3

MAYO
©2002

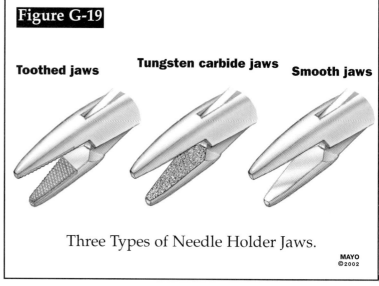

Figure G-19

Toothed jaws   Tungsten carbide jaws   Smooth jaws

Three Types of Needle Holder Jaws.

MAYO
©2002

G. Surgical Instruments

7. Hemostat

The hemostat is a clamp designed to grasp blood vessels prior to cauterization or ligation. The instrument is held much like a needle holder. The hemostat is held in the palm of the hand with the thumb and fourth finger in the rings (holes) of the handle **(Figure G-20)**.

When clamping a blood vessel to stop bleeding you should clamp just the blood vessel and avoid clamping excessive surrounding tissue **(Figure G-21A)**. A blood vessel is clamped with the curved tips of two hemostats **facing** each other **(Figure G-21B)**. The vessel is cut between the two hemostats **(Figure G-21C)**.

Hemostasis is achieved by tying suture around the blood vessel below the clamp **(Figure G-21D)**. This tying of suture around a blood vessel is called a vessel ligature.

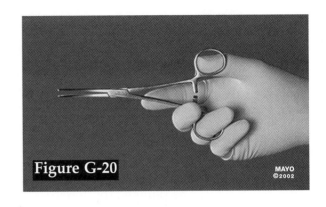

Figure G-20

MAYO
©2002

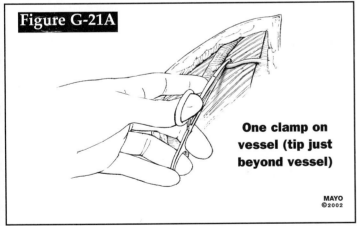

Figure G-21A

One clamp on vessel (tip just beyond vessel)

MAYO
©2002

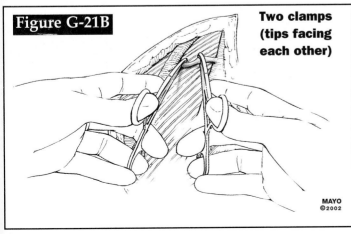

Figure G-21B

Two clamps (tips facing each other)

MAYO
©2002

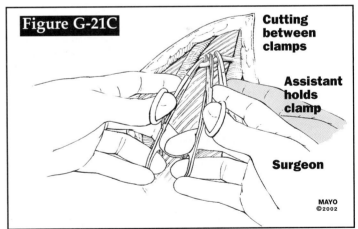

Figure G-21C

Cutting between clamps

Assistant holds clamp

Surgeon

MAYO
©2002

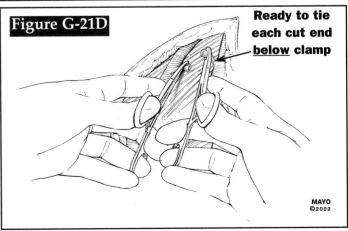

Figure G-21D

Ready to tie each cut end <u>below</u> clamp

MAYO
©2002

G. Surgical Instruments

8. Suction

There are various suction instruments used to remove fluids and blood from the surgical field **(Figures G,22-23)**. Some suctions are continuous while others are intermittent. Continuous suction does not have a side port and produces a sustained and continuous suction effect **(Figure G-24)**. The intermittent suctions have a side port hole that can be plugged (occluded) which allows the suction effect to occur. When the side port hole is unplugged, or open, the suction is turned off **(Figure G-24)**.

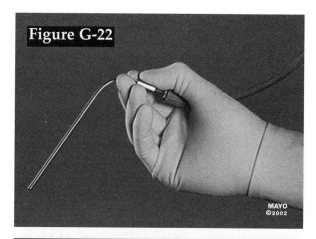

Figure G-22

Figure G-23

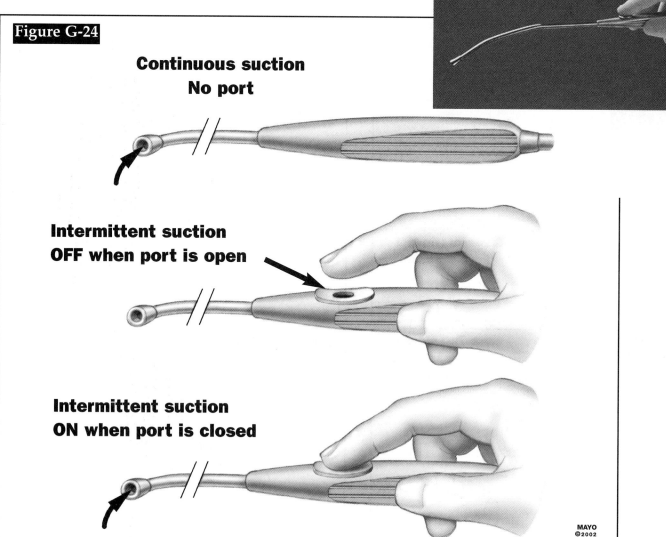

Figure G-24

**Continuous suction
No port**

**Intermittent suction
OFF when port is open**

**Intermittent suction
ON when port is closed**

G. Surgical Instruments

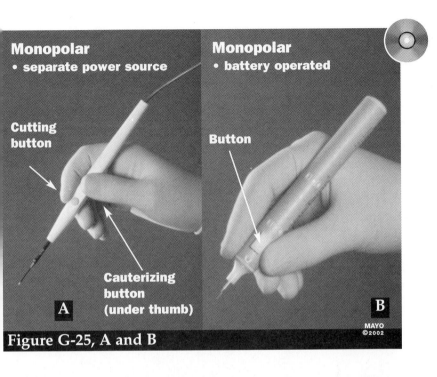

Monopolar
• separate power source

Cutting button

Cauterizing button (under thumb)

A

Monopolar
• battery operated

Button

B

MAYO
©2002

Figure G-25, A and B

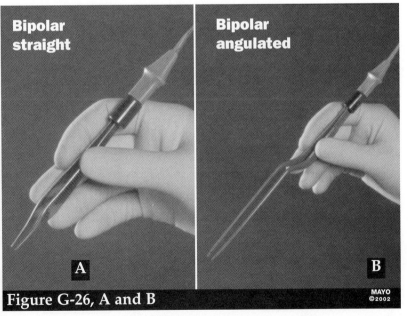

Bipolar straight

A

Bipolar angulated

B

MAYO
©2002

Figure G-26, A and B

9. Cautery

A cautery is an instrument used to coagulate (cauterize) and cut tissue. Cautery is an electrical current which coagulates the blood vessels to arrest bleeding. There are two types of cautery: monopolar and bipolar. The monopolar cautery generates more heat than the bipolar cautery.

a. Monopolar cautery is a cautery with one pole. The current can be used to both cauterize (coagulate) and to cut tissues **(Figure G-25, A)**. There are two types. One is powered by a separate electrical source while the other is battery operated. Both types are disposable **(Figure G-25, A and B)**. Press the button to activate the electric current. Cautery is rarely used to cut skin. Occasionally the cautery will be used to incise and cauterize the deeper tissues for speed and hemostasis.

b. Bipolar cautery is a cautery with two poles, one on each side of a forceps-like instrument. Basically there are two types of bipolar cautery. One is straight **(Figure G-26, A)** and the other is angulated **(Figure G-26, B)**. The tissue that is grasped in the forceps of the bipolar cautery is cauterized. Using a bipolar cautery is more precise and results in less transmission of heat to surrounding tissues. A bipolar cautery is usually activated by a foot pedal.

G. Surgical Instruments

10. Suture Scissors

Suture scissors are used to cut suture. You will probably use the suture scissors as the first instrument of your initial surgical experience (**Figure G-27**).

Sutures that are buried are left within the body. These sutures are usually cut on the knot (**Figure G-28**). Cutting on the knot cuts the tails off the ends of the suture. To accomplish this, you slide the suture scissors down the suture until the knot is felt just under the blades of the suture scissors. Then the scissors are turned slightly so **you** can **see** the knot and then cut the suture flush on the knot (**Figure G-28**).

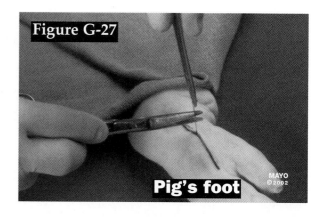

Figure G-27

Pig's foot

MAYO ©2002

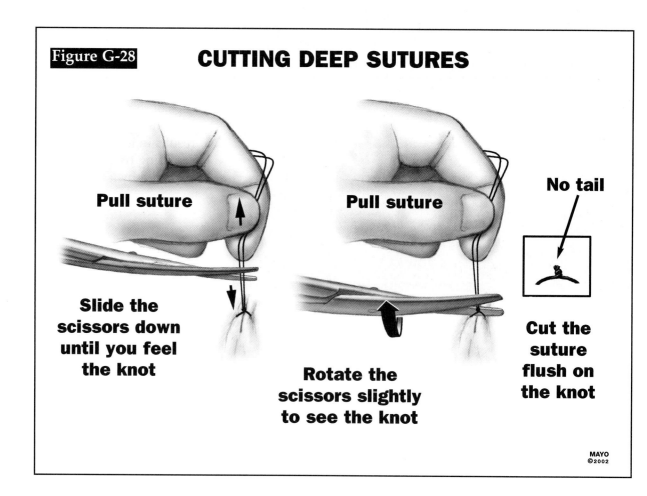

Figure G-28   **CUTTING DEEP SUTURES**

Pull suture

Slide the scissors down until you feel the knot

Pull suture

Rotate the scissors slightly to see the knot

No tail

Cut the suture flush on the knot

MAYO ©2002

G. Surgical Instruments

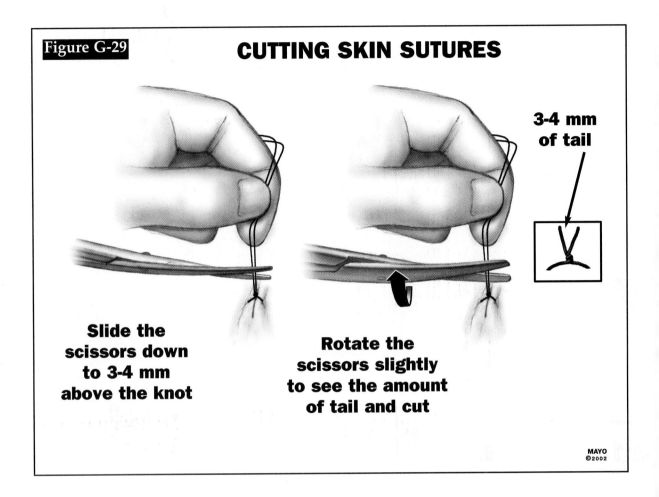

Figure G-29

CUTTING SKIN SUTURES

Slide the
scissors down
to 3-4 mm
above the knot

Rotate the
scissors slightly
to see the amount
of tail and cut

3-4 mm
of tail

MAYO
©2002

When a tail is to be left behind, especially on skin sutures, slide the scissors down the suture to the appropriate tail length, turn, and then cut. This turning of the scissors allows the surgical assistant to visualize the knot and the amount of tail that will be left behind (**Figure G-29**). This technique ensures the proper length of the tail that is left behind. Usually an appropriate tail length for skin sutures is about three or four millimeters.

Why is a tail left? Leaving three to four millimeters of a suture tail helps prevent loosening, knot slippage, and undoing of the sutures. Grasping the tail with forceps also facilitates suture removal postoperatively. To remove a suture you lift the suture with a forceps, cut with scissors and remove the suture, usually 5 - 14 days after surgery and this depends on the surgical site (location). Facial incisions heal more rapidly than abdominal incisions and therefore facial sutures are removed earlier than abdominal sutures.

G. Surgical Instruments

11. Towel Clip

A towel clip is used to hold surgical drapes and towels together. It is held like a hemostat (**Figure G-30**). During draping of the patient to prepare the surgical field, drapes are held in place most often with towel clips.

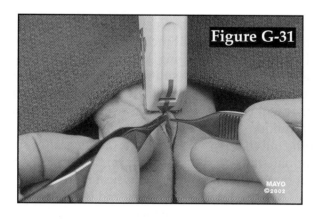

Figure G-30

12. Staple Gun

The hand-held disposable staple gun is used to apply metal staples to close the skin (**Figure G-31**). This is especially useful for rapid closure of many incisions. Staples are **never** used in the face.

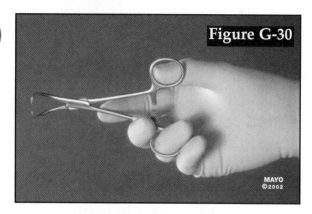

Figure G-31

13. Additional Equipment Used in Operating Room

a. Laryngoscope
Instrument used to examine the larynx and introduce an endotracheal tube into the trachea during general anesthesia (**Figure G-32**).

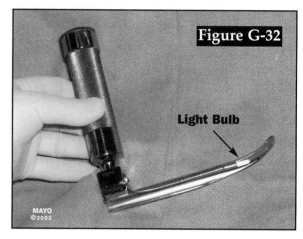

Figure G-32

Light Bulb

b. Endotracheal Tube
Used to administer anesthetic gases. The inflated baloon secures the tube in the trachea (**Figure G-33**).

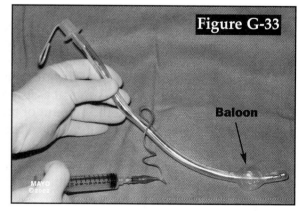

Figure G-33

Baloon

G. Surgical Instruments

c. Oral Airway
Used to keep the jaw and tongue from falling back and blocking the airway. This is inserted as the patient is waking up ("comes out") from general anesthesia **(Figure G-34)**.

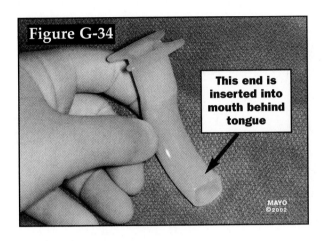

This end is inserted into mouth behind tongue

d. Endoscopes
"Scopes" used to magnify and visualize a specific surgical field **(Figure G-35A-C)**.

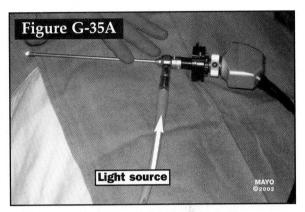

Light source

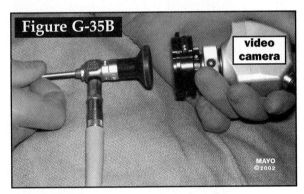

video camera

Attaching video camera to endoscope

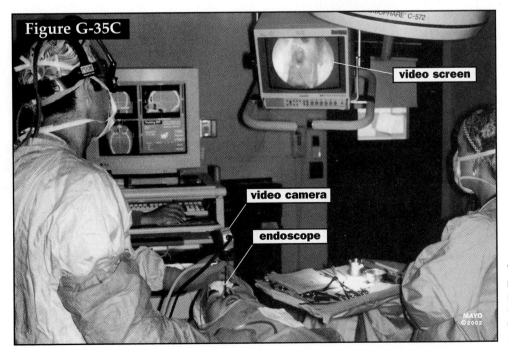

video screen

video camera

endoscope

Viewing interior of nose on video screen with endoscope and attached camera during surgery.

G. Surgical Instruments

e. Anesthesia Cart

The anesthesia cart is used as a compact site for all the specialized equipment used when surgery is carried out under general anesthesia **(Figure G-36)**.

1. Reservoir bag

2. Bellows

3. Air/N20/O2 flow dials

4. Volatile anesthetics

5. Ventilator

6. Monitor for vital signs

7. Mass spectrometer

8. Suction

9. Hoses to/from patient

10. Exchanging system

11. Inspiratory/ expiratory valves

12. Call system

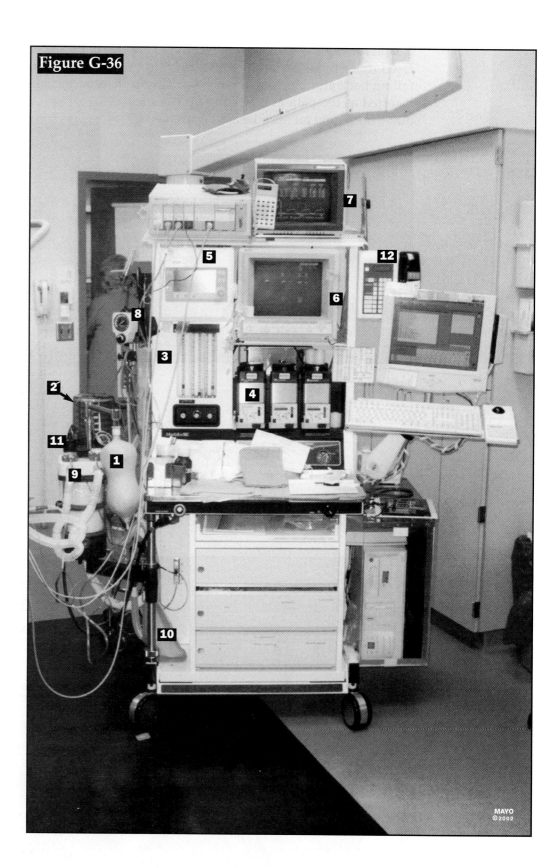

Figure G-36

MAYO
©2002

G. Surgical Instruments

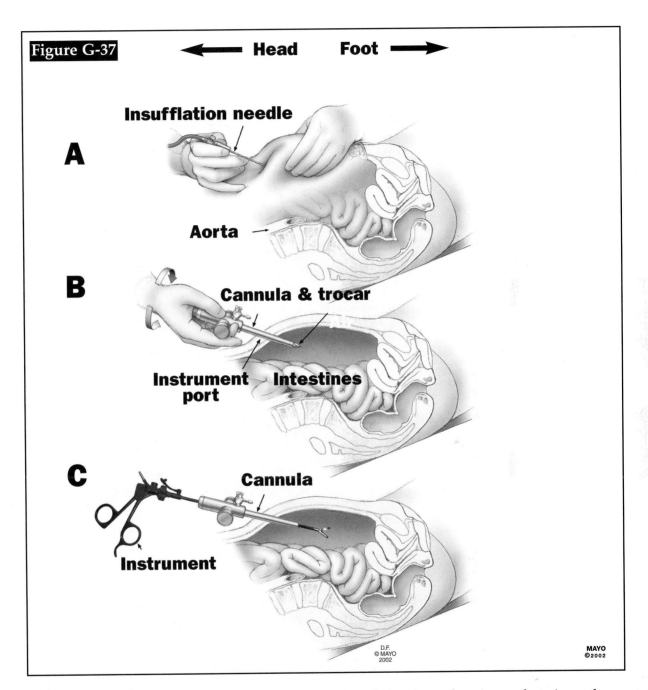

Figure G-37

← Head Foot →

A Insufflation needle

Aorta

B Cannula & trocar

Instrument port Intestines

C Cannula

Instrument

D.F. © MAYO 2002

MAYO ©2002

f. Some Endoscopic Instruments Used In General Surgery

In **Figure G-37** you can understand the process by which the abdominal contents may be exposed, viewed and operated upon using an endoscopic, minimally invasive approach and technique. In **Figure G-37A**, the abdominal wall is grasped and retracted away from the underlying abdominal contents while an insufflation needle penetrates into the peritoneal cavity so that air can be introduced pushing the intestines aside. This pneumoperitoneum (air in peritoneal cavity) provides the tension which allows the cannula and trocar **(Figure G-37B)** to produce a hole or **"instrument port"** through which endoscopic instruments can be introduced (through the cannula) without injury to vital organs **(Figure G-37C)**.

G. Surgical Instruments

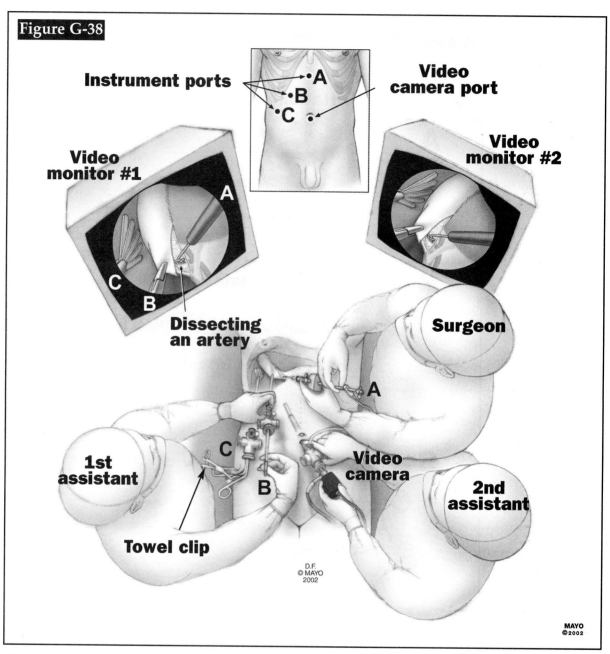

Figure G-38

- Instrument ports — •A, •B, •C
- Video camera port
- Video monitor #1
- Video monitor #2
- A
- C
- B
- Dissecting an artery
- Surgeon
- 1st assistant
- C
- B
- Video camera
- 2nd assistant
- Towel clip
- A

D.F.
© MAYO
2002

MAYO
©2002

Figure G-38 demonstrates the **instrument port** sites **(A,B,C)** and **video camera port** site through which endoscopic abdominal surgery may be carried out. The surgeon views video monitor #1 while he dissects an artery through instrument port A. The first assistant operating through instrument port B produces traction with a grasping instrument while viewing video monitor #2. A fan retractor is held in place with a towel clip at instrument port C. The second assistant maneuvers the video camera while watching video monitor #1.

Figure G-39 illustrates only a few of the many instruments used in endoscopic abdominal surgery.

G. Surgical Instruments

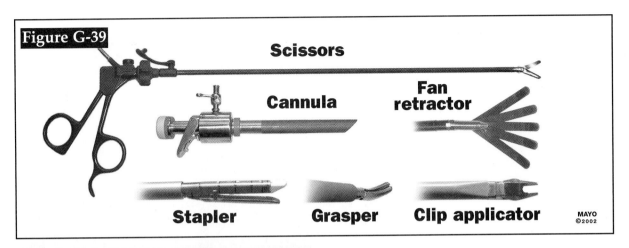

Figure G-39

Scissors

Cannula

Fan retractor

Stapler

Grasper

Clip applicator

MAYO ©2002

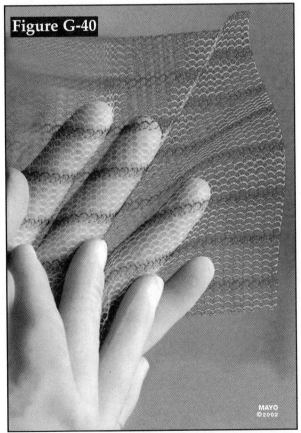

Figure G-40

MAYO ©2002

g. Polypropylene (Prolene®) Mesh
This is a synthetic surgical mesh that is non-absorbable and flexible for use in hernia repair either by laparoscopic or open surgical approach **(Figure G-40)**.

G. Surgical Instruments

Quiz

Fill in the shaded blanks! See page 17, Figure C-7 for the correct answers.

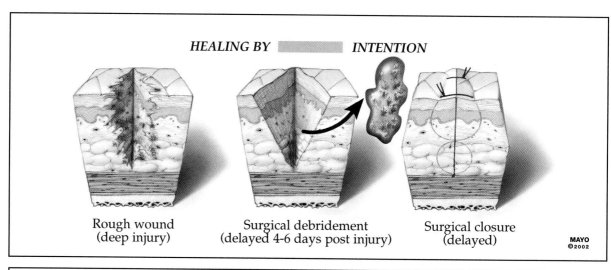

HEALING BY ▨▨▨▨ INTENTION

Rough wound
(deep injury)

Surgical debridement
(delayed 4-6 days post injury)

Surgical closure
(delayed)

MAYO
©2002

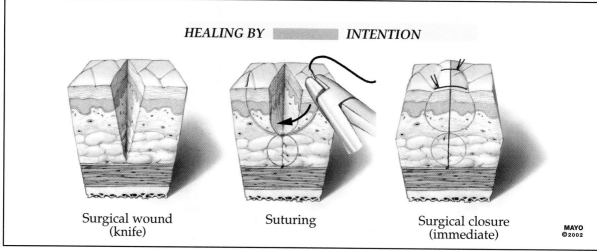

HEALING BY ▨▨▨▨ INTENTION

Surgical wound
(knife)

Suturing

Surgical closure
(immediate)

MAYO
©2002

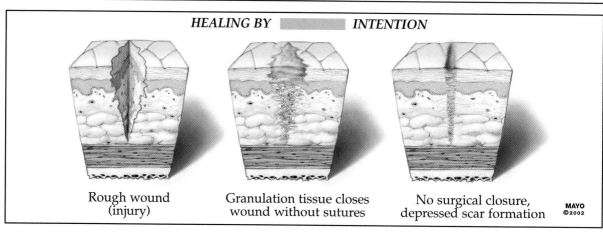

HEALING BY ▨▨▨▨ INTENTION

Rough wound
(injury)

Granulation tissue closes
wound without sutures

No surgical closure,
depressed scar formation

MAYO
©2002

Quiz

?

Fill in the shaded blanks and answer the questions below! See page 49, Figure G-37 for the correct answers.

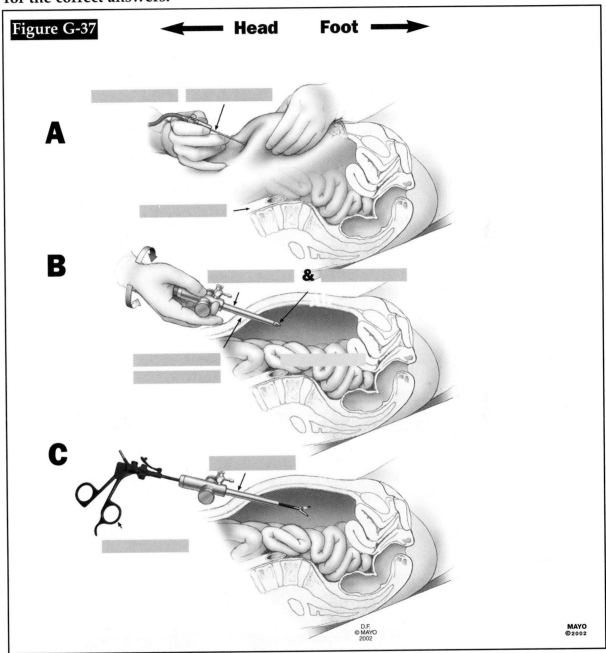

Figure G-37 ← **Head   Foot** →

A

B

C

D.F.
© MAYO
2002

MAYO
©2002

1. What is the purpose of the insufflation needle?

2. What is the purpose of producing a pneumoperitoneum?

3. After removal of the _____ you can pass an instrument through the cannula.

Quiz

Fill in the shaded blanks! See page 35, Figure G-5 for the correct answers.

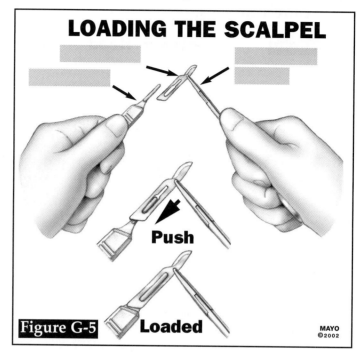

Fill in the shaded blanks! See page 45 Figure G-29 for the correct answers.

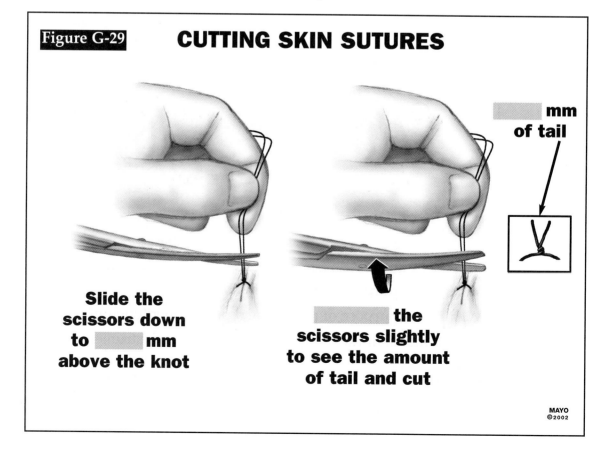

H. Sutures, Needles and Knots

1. Introduction

Sutures are materials used to close wounds. Ligatures are materials used to close blood vessels. Sutures and ligatures were used by both the Egyptians and Syrians two thousand years B.C. Suturing was performed even in the time of Hippocrates. Sheep intestines were first mentioned as suture material in the writings of Galen, the Roman physician. The first reports of suturing abdominal wounds appeared in the work of Rhazes, the Arabian surgeon, in approximately 800 A.D. As a surgeon you will hear the term catgut. This is actually a misnomer because it does not refer to cats or guts. Catgut is derived from the Arabic word "kitgut," which refers to the strings of a violin.

After the introduction of anesthetics in the middle of the 19th century and the use of antiseptics by Joseph Lister in 1865, the art and science of surgery progressed rapidly. The development of sutures and suturing techniques paralleled the development of surgery. The early 1950s heralded the introduction of the individually packed, pre-sterilized suture material.

How do you proceed to close a wound? A wound is usually closed in anatomic layers. The one exception is the wound of the eyelid where the skin and underlying orbicularis oculi muscle layers are extremely thin and can be closed as one layer. Most wounds are closed at each specific anatomic structure or layer. For example, the incised muscle layers, subcutaneous tissues, and skin are closed separately. The muscle layers and the subcutaneous layers are usually closed with buried, absorbable suture. The skin is usually closed with a non-absorbable suture. In high tension wounds, which are wounds that are difficult to bring together, longer lasting absorbable or permanent subcutaneous suture may be required to prevent wound breakdown.

Prior to starting the wound closure, **under-mining** the skin and soft tissues is done to relieve tension at the wound edges. This allows the wound to be approximated and closed without tension. Undermining of one or two centimeters from the wound edge will decrease wound closing tension. The undermining of the soft tissues beyond and below the incision can be done with either a scalpel or scissors. Undermining beyond two centimeters from the wound edge **does not** further decrease wound closing tension. As a young surgeon, you should begin undermining with scissors. This is because you can undermine quickly and safely with the dissection scissors.

What do you need to know about suture materials? Some of the important factors regarding suturing material choice for surgery include diameter, tensile strength, tissue reactivity, the ease of handling the suture material, the facility for tying and maintaining knots, plus the absorption of the sutures by the body.

2. Suture Materials

There are a great variety of suture materials, suture sizes, and needle sizes available. Suture materials are divided into absorbable and non-absorbable types. We have tried to simplify the entire topic of suture materials by using the table format to summarize the important points. First, some basic concepts.

The primary use for sutures is to maintain and hold the wound together in approximation as the tissues heal and the tensile strength increases. See **Table H-1** which demonstrates the increasing tensile strength of the healing wound after injury. The healing wound can be affected by the type of suture material, the suture technique and the tension on the wounded tissue produced by the sutures themselves. In general, suture material should be strong (tensile strength) yet easy to use. The surgical knots that are tied must remain secure and induce minimal tissue reactivity. This tissue reactivity refers to the inflammatory response the suture itself causes because it acts like a foreign body.

H. Sutures, Needles and Knots

Table H-1 Increasing Tensile Strength of the Wound After Injury

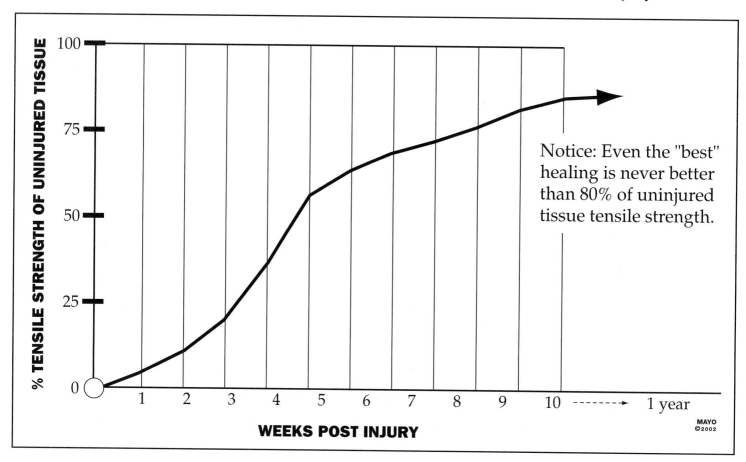

Notice: Even the "best" healing is never better than 80% of uninjured tissue tensile strength.

MAYO
©2002

Tensile strength is low at first but increases from 10% at 2 weeks to 40% by one month. It reaches about 80% of original tensile strength after 10 weeks.

H. Sutures, Needles and Knots

a. Absorbable sutures

Absorbable sutures are dissolved by the body and do not require removal **(Table H-2)**. Absorbable sutures come in polyfilament (braided) and monofilament (unbraided) sutures. Each have various half-lives and strengths. The most common absorbable sutures include gut which is a natural material and various synthetic materials including polyglycolic acid (Dexon®), polyglactin 9-10 (Vicryl®), polydioxanone (PDS®), and polyglicaprone 25 (Monocryl®).

Table H-2
ABSORBABLE Suture Materials

NAME	SURGICAL HANDLING (Ease of tying)	TENSILE STRENGTH (Strength remaining)	KNOT SECURITY (How well it holds a knot)	TISSIE REACTIVITY (How much inflammation it causes)	ABSORPTION TIME (About how long it lasts)	CLINICAL USES
NATURAL MATERIAL						
SURGICAL GUT **(plain)** Polyfilament	Fair	Poor at 1 week	Poor	Major	1-2 weeks	Subcutaneaous closure
SURGICAL GUT **(chromic)** Polyfilament	Fair	Poor at 3 weeks	Poor	Moderate	2-3 weeks	Subcutaneaous closure
SURGICAL GUT **(fast absorbing)** Polyfilament	Fair	0% at 1 week	Poor	Moderate	1 week	Skin closure
SYNTHETIC MATERIAL						
POLYGLACTIN 910 **(Vicryl®)** Polyfilament	Good	50% at 3 weeks	Good	Minor	2-3 months	Subcutaneous closure
POLYGLYCOLIC **(Dexon®)** Polyfilament	Good	50% at 3 weeks	Good	Minor	2-3 months	Subcutaneous closure, ligature of vessels
POLYDIOXANONE **(PDS®)** Monofilament	Fair	50% at 4 weeks	Good	Minor	6 months	Contaminated subcutaneous closure, (high tension closures)
POLYGLECAPRONE 25 **(Monocryl®)** Monofilament	Good	40% at 2 weeks	Good	Minor	3 months	Intradermal (also called subcuticular or intracuticular)

H. Sutures, Needles and Knots

Gut, Dexon®, and Vicryl® are polyfilament sutures, which means that they are braided together for increased strength. While the polyfilament sutures have the advantage of being braided for strength, they have the disadvantage of a "wick effect" that can allow bacterial penetration between the braids of the suture. Monofilament sutures are not braided. Both collagen and surgical gut sutures can be plain or chromic. Chromatizing means that the half-life of the suture will be extended (by a chemical process) so the suture will stay in place longer. This facilitates wound healing before the sutures lose their tensile strength and fall apart.

b. Non-absorbable suture
Non-absorbable sutures are not dissolved by the body and do require removal **(Table H-3)**. Silk is a braided suture and for this reason may cause microabscesses along the wound edge and is rarely used for epidermal (skin) closure. Nylon and polypropylene are most commonly used for skin closure as well as for buried and long-term "permanent" suture placement. Stainless steel is used to close the sternum of the chest but has few other uses because of its difficult handling properties. Stainless steel staples are excellent for skin closure.

Table H-3
NON-ABSORBABLE Suture Materials

NAME	STYLE	SURGICAL HANDLING (Ease of tying)	TENSILE STRENGTH (Strength remaining)	KNOT SECURITY (How well it holds a knot)	TISSIE REACTIVITY (How much inflamation it causes)	CLINICAL USES
NATURAL MATERIAL						
SILK	Braided or Twisted	Excellent	0% at 1 year	Good	Moderate	Ligature of vessels
SYNTHETIC MATERIAL						
NYLON						
Ethilon®	Monofilament	Fair-Good	20% at 1 year	Fair	Minor	Skin closure
Dermalon®	Monofilament	Fair-Good	20% at 1 year	Fair	Minor	Skin closure
Nurolon®	Braided	Fair-Good	20% at 1 year	Fair	Minor	Skin closure
POLYPROPYLENE **Prolene®**	Monofilament	Fair-Good	Permanent	Poor	Minor	Skin closure
POLYESTER **Mersilene®**	Braided	Very good	Permanent	Good	Minor	Subcutaneous closure
Ethibond®	Braided	Very good	Permanent	Good	Minor	
STAINLESS STEEL	Monofilament Braided or Twisted	Poor*	Permanent	Good	Almost none	Bone, sternum, jaw, tendon, etc.

MAYO
©2002

H. Sutures, Needles and Knots

Table H-4

The lower the suture size number, the larger (thicker) the diameter and the higher (greater, stronger) the tensile strength.

The higher the suture size number, the smaller (thinner) the diameter and the lower (less, weaker) the tensile strength.

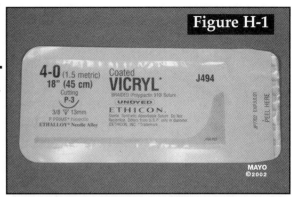

Figure H-1

Suture Size	Suture Diameter	Tensile Strength
1-0	Larger (thicker)	High (greater, stronger)
2-00		
3-000		
4-0000		
5-00000		
6-000000		
7-0000000		
8-00000000		
9-000000000		
10-0000000000		
11-00000000000	Smaller (thinner)	Lower (less, weaker)

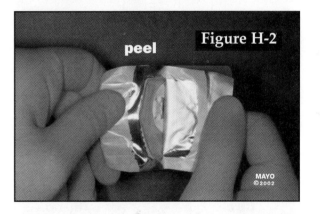

Figure H-2

Figure H-3

MAYO
©2002

Conventional suture package and opening technique to expose inner package with needle and suture are shown **(Figures H, 1-4)**.

It is important to know how to read the suture package labels. This basic information is found in **Figures H, 5-7**.

Some generalizations can be made regarding the best suture choice for the skin closure of a particular body location. **Table H-5** shows suture selection typical for each site. You should always consider using **ABSORBABLE** sutures in children or the non-compliant adult. Rarely, high tension cutaneous (skin) wounds are closed with 0 or 2-0 sutures. These may be utilized as bolster sutures to help relieve tension on large abdominal wounds.

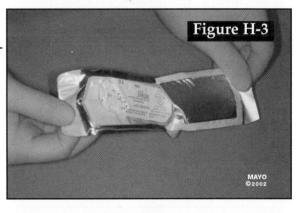

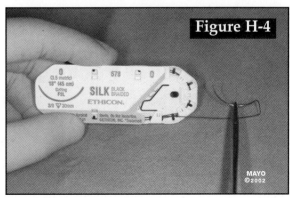

Figure H-4

H. Sutures, Needles and Knots

HOW TO READ THE SUTURE PACKAGE

Peelable Foil Pack
Synthetic absorbables only

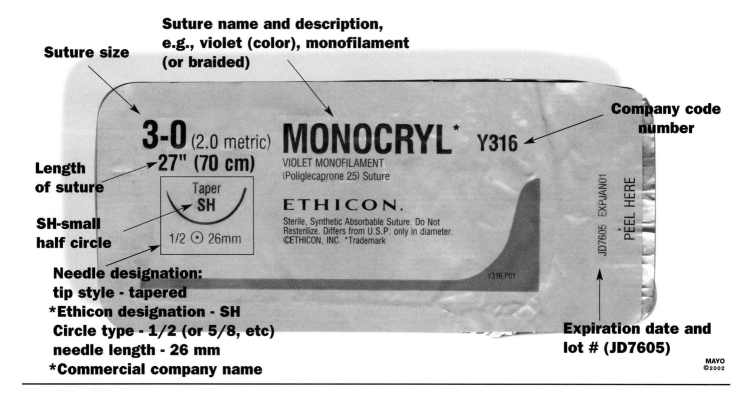

Suture name and description,
e.g., violet (color), monofilament
(or braided)

Suture size

Company code
number

Length
of suture

SH-small
half circle

Needle designation:
tip style - tapered
*Ethicon designation - SH
Circle type - 1/2 (or 5/8, etc)
needle length - 26 mm
*Commercial company name

Expiration date and
lot # (JD7605)

MAYO
©2002

Figure H-6

Internal Package
Read the same way

(called "relay package")

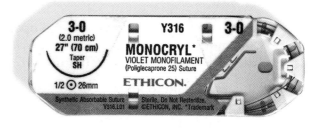

MAYO
©2002

Figure H-7

Conventional Package
Read the same way

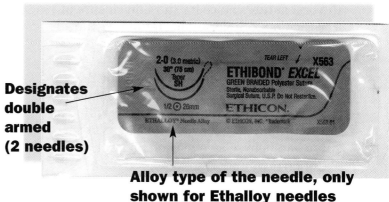

Designates
double
armed
(2 needles)

Alloy type of the needle, only
shown for Ethalloy needles

MAYO
©2002

H. Sutures, Needles and Knots

Table H-5
Typical Suture Choices (Suture Size and Suture Material)

SITE	DEEP LAYERS (SUTURE SIZE)	SUTURE MATERIALS	SKIN LAYER (SUTURE SIZE)	SUTURE MATERIALS
SCALP	2-0 to 4-0	Absorbable	4-0 to 5-0	Nylon, polypropylene, or staples
EYELID	5-0 to 7-0	"	6-0 to 7-0	Nylon, polypropylene, plain gut
FACE	3-0 to 5-0	"	5-0 to 6-0	Nylon, polypropylene, plain gut
NECK	2-0 to 4-0	"	4-0 to 5-0	Nylon, polypropylene, plain gut, or staples
TRUNK	2-0 to 3-0	"	2-0 to 4-0	Nylon, polypropylene, or staples
LIMBS	2-0 to 4-0	"	3-0 to 5-0	Nylon, polypropylene, or staples
HANDS AND FEET	3-0 to 5-0	"	4-0 to 5-0	Nylon, polypropylene, or staples
SOLES OF FEET	2-0 to 4-0	"	2-0 to 4-0	Nylon, polypropylene, or staples

3. Choosing a Surgical Needle

The main purpose of the surgical needle is to pierce the wound edges so the suture material can approximate the tissues and close the wound.

The main considerations for needle selection are:

1. Type of tissues to be closed.
2. Curvature of needle is selected based on the space of operative field.

Needle sharpness and ductility (refers to a needle's bending and resistance to breaking under a given amount of stress when piercing tissues) are both important. The taper point and fine silicone coating of the needle enhances its initial penetration and reduces drag and resistance as the needle passes repeatedly through the tissues being repaired. A **taper point needle** is useful for closure of delicate structures like mucosal structures **(Figure H-10A)**. For thick skin usually a **conventional cutting needle** is best **(Figure H-11A)**.

Care must still be taken to avoid excessive tearing through tissue using the conventional cutting needle since the cutting surface is on inner edge.

Surgical needles are designed to pass suture through various tissues with as minimal tissue trauma as possible. The needles are composed

H. Sutures, Needles and Knots

of three specific parts. The basic components of a surgical needle include: 1) the point, 2) the body, and 3) the eye **(Figure H-8).**

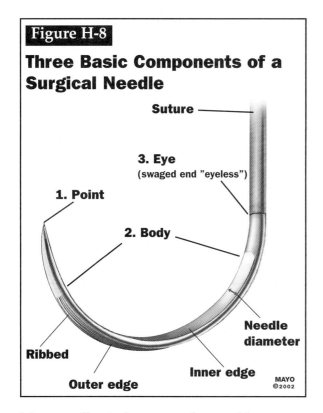

Figure H-8

Three Basic Components of a Surgical Needle

Suture

3. Eye
(swaged end "eyeless")

1. Point

2. Body

Ribbed

Needle diameter

Outer edge

Inner edge

MAYO
©2002

Most needles today are eyeless and have a swaged end so the suture does not have to be threaded. The other needle types include the closed eye and French (open) eye needle **(Figure H-9).**

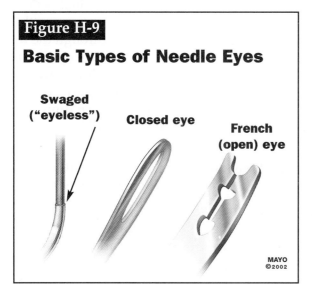

Figure H-9

Basic Types of Needle Eyes

Swaged
("eyeless")

Closed eye

French
(open) eye

MAYO
©2002

4. Common Needle Types

Common needles used in surgery are (1) tapered **(Figure H-10A,B)** and (2) cutting **(Figure H-11A,B).** The tapered needle has a pointed end, but the rest of the needle itself is a smooth, rounded tube with no cutting edges.

a. Tapered Needles

The tapered needle minimizes tissue trauma. It is commonly used in general surgery for closure of mucosal incisions, like those in the stomach or small intestine.

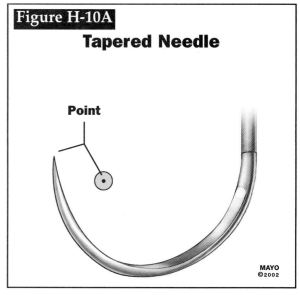

Figure H-10A

Tapered Needle

Point

MAYO
©2002

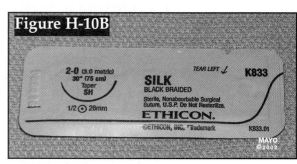

Figure H-10B

2-0 (3.0 metric)
30" (75 cm)
Taper
SH

1/2 ⊙ 26mm

TEAR LEFT

SILK
BLACK BRAIDED

Sterile, Nonabsorbable Surgical
Suture, U.S.P. Do Not Resterilize.

ETHICON.

©ETHICON, INC. *Trademark

K833

K833.01

MAYO
©2002

H. Sutures, Needles and Knots

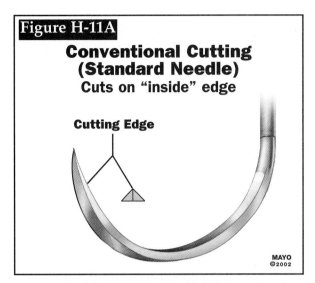

Figure H-11A

Conventional Cutting (Standard Needle)
Cuts on "inside" edge

Cutting Edge

MAYO
©2002

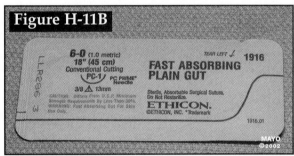

Figure H-11B

6-0 (1.0 metric)
18" (45 cm)
Conventional Cutting
PC-1 PC PRIME Needle
3/8 △ 13mm

TEAR LEFT ↙ 1916

FAST ABSORBING PLAIN GUT

Sterile, Absorbable Surgical Suture,
Do Not Resterilize.

ETHICON.
©ETHICON, INC. *Trademark

1916.01

MAYO
©2002

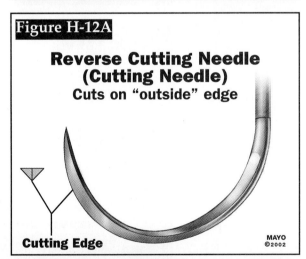

Figure H-12A

Reverse Cutting Needle (Cutting Needle)
Cuts on "outside" edge

Cutting Edge

MAYO
©2002

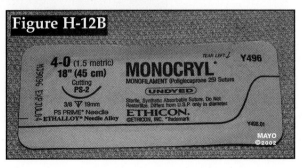

Figure H-12B

4-0 (1.5 metric)
18" (45 cm)
Cutting
PS-2
3/8 ▽ 19mm
PS PRIME Needle
ETHALLOY Needle Alloy

TEAR LEFT ↙ Y496

MONOCRYL
MONOFILAMENT (Poliglecaprone 25) Suture

UNDYED

Sterile, Synthetic Absorbable Suture, Do Not
Resterilize. Differs from U.S.P. only in diameter

ETHICON.
©ETHICON, INC. *Trademark

Y496.01

MAYO
©2002

b. Cutting Needles

The cutting needle has a sharp end and sharp edges (**Figure H-11 A,B**). Therefore, the entire needle acts as a cutting instrument. The cutting needle is commonly used for subcutaneous, intradermal, and cutaneous (skin) closure. Because of the sharp point and sharp edges, this needle is more amenable to cutting through tougher tissues.

1. Conventional cutting needles
The conventional cutting needles have the opposing cutting edges plus a third cutting edge on the inner (concave) side, which is useful for cutting through tough resistant tissues like skin (**Figure H-11 A,B**).

There are special plastic surgery needles that are conventional cutting needles. These needles are excellent for delicate facial surgery because of the narrow point, narrow diameter with a fine taper so soft tissue can be easily penetrated.

The body of the needle is flattened which facilitates needle stability with the needle holder.

2. Reverse cutting needles
Sometimes referred to simply as "cutting", this needle's cutting edge is on the (outer, convex) side.

These needles were designed to penetrate very tough tissues easily and without bending or breaking the needle. These tough tissues include skin, oral mucosa, tendon sheaths, **periosteum**, and other tough thick tissues. These reverse cutting needles are superior for cosmetic ophthalmic (eye) surgery because they cause minimal trauma and minimal scar tissue formation which is paramount in these surgical situations. The reverse cutting needle has the sharp two opposing cutting edges for tissue entry and, in addition, has a third cutting edge on the outer (convex) curve of the needle making it stronger than the same rigid conventional cutting needle (**Figure H-12 A,B**).

H. Sutures, Needles and Knots

Using the reverse cutting needle, there is less chance for tearing the tissue during the needle pass. In addition, the hole left by the needle leaves a wider amount of tissue against which to tie the suture.

C. Blunt Needles
These needles were designed especially for liver and kidney surgery **(Figure H-13 A,B)**. While the point of the needle is blunt the upper 2/3 of the body is usually flat to allow the needle holder (driver) to grasp the needle body firmly.

d. Special Rules for Handling of Needles During Surgery

1. When a needle breaks you must find all the pieces.

2. Discard needles in "sharps container".

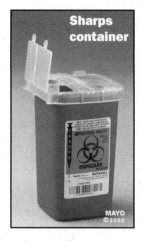

3. Avoid needle sticks by using a "non pass back" technique. This is also called the "non-transfer technique," where the surgeon places the needle holder down on the field so the scrub nurse can pick it up.

5. In the "pass" technique, the scrub nurse "passes" the needle holder to the surgeon with needlepoint toward the surgeons thumb. This prevents excess wrist motion while holding the free end of suture which prevents dragging the suture across the sterile field **(Figure H-14 A,B)**.

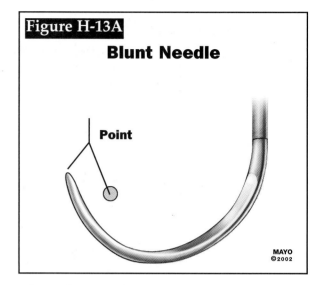

Figure H-13A

Blunt Needle

Point

MAYO
©2002

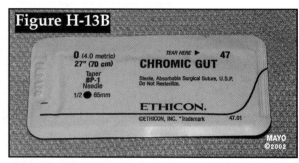

Figure H-13B

0 (4.0 metric)
27" (70 cm)
Taper
BP-1
Needle
1/2 ● 65mm

TEAR HERE ▶   47
CHROMIC GUT
Sterile, Absorbable Surgical Suture, U.S.P.
Do Not Resterilize.

ETHICON.
©ETHICON, INC. *Trademark   47.01

MAYO
©2002

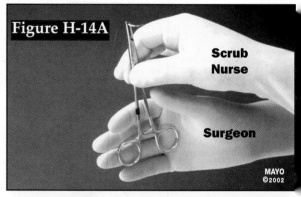

Figure H-14A

Scrub Nurse

Surgeon

MAYO
©2002

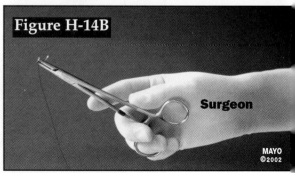

Figure H-14B

Surgeon

MAYO
©2002

H. Sutures, Needles and Knots

e. Common Manufacturers Letter Designations for Needles.
There are manufacturer letters associated with their needles. The most common needles used in the USA are either from Ethicon or Davis and Geck.

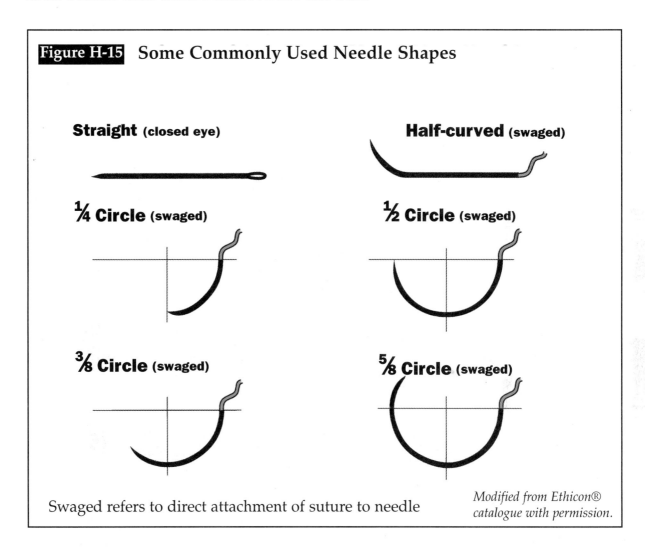

Figure H-15 Some Commonly Used Needle Shapes

Straight (closed eye)

Half-curved (swaged)

¼ Circle (swaged)

½ Circle (swaged)

⅜ Circle (swaged)

⅝ Circle (swaged)

Swaged refers to direct attachment of suture to needle

Modified from Ethicon® catalogue with permission.

Some <u>Davis & Geck</u> needles have the following designations:

1. CE (cutting and E refers to 3/8 of a circle in curvature)

2. SBE (slim blade) reverse cutting and slim body

3. DP (diamond point)

4. SC (skin closure) reverse and standard cutting

5. PRE (premium)

The needles themselves come in various shapes and sizes depending upon their use. Most needles are curved, although straight needles are available for a variety of applications. See **Figures H-15** and **H-16** for some commonly used needle shapes and needles.

H. Sutures, Needles and Knots

Figure H-16 **Some Commonly Used Needles**

PRECISION POINT

-Reverse Cutting ▽ (also called "Cutting")
3/8 Circle:

P-3

PS-2

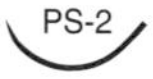

(P = Plastic)
(PS = Plastic Surgery)

1/2 Circle:

OS-2

(OS = Orthopedic Surgery)

- Conventional Cutting △ (also called "Standard")
3/8 Circle: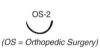

CFS

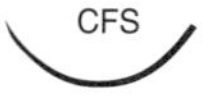

PRECISION COSMETIC

- Conventional Cutting △

3/8 Circle:

PC-1

PC-3

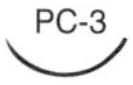

Some Ethicon needles have the following designations:

1. FS (for skin)
2. P (plastic)
3. PS (plastic surgery)
4. CPS (conventional plastic surgery)
5. PC (precision cosmetic)

The PC is the needle of choice for skin closure since it is a standard cutting needle which allows penetration and reduced resistance passing through the skin.

6. BP (blunt point) - for liver and kidney
7. SH (small half circle) - for bowel
8. CT (circle taper) - for fascia
9. SC (Nasal Septal Cartilage

MICROPOINT

-Reverse Cutting ▽ (also called "Cutting")
3/8 Circle:

G-6

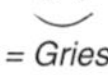

(G = Grieshaber)

-Spatula �⌣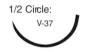

1/2 Circle:

OPS-5

(OPS = Orthopedic Plastic)

TAPER CUT ▽

3/8 Circle:

CC-1

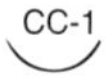

(CC = Calcified Coronary)

1/2 Circle:

V-37

(Sternum closure and orthopedics)

TAPER POINT

1/2 Circle:

SH

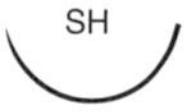

*(SH = Small Half circle,
for G.I. surgery)*

CT-1

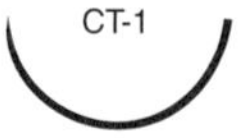

*(CT = Circle Taper),
for fascia closures*

STRAIGHT ▽

SC-1

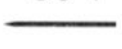

(SC = Septal Cartilage)

BLUNT POINT ●

1/2 Circle:

BP-1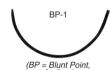

*(BP = Blunt Point,
for liver)*

Modified from Ethicon® catalogue with permission.

H. Sutures, Needles and Knots

5. Knot Tying

So now you are ready to tie surgical knots. Try to remember back to first learning to tie your shoes as a toddler! At times the skill will come slowly. But once mastered, surgical knot tying will never be forgotten. Please liberally reference the CD-ROM Disc 1 portion of this course during this section. The combination of both still photos, animation and practice should help acquire these skills.

a. Two-Hand Tie - Right Handed Surgeon
The two-hand tie is the first type of tie that should be learned. Why? Because it is the most useful. This tie gives the best knot security, especially when compared with the one-hand tie. You must master the two-hand tie early because tying will be one of the first tasks you will be asked to perform as an assistant in surgery. The hand position varies depending upon whether you are a **right-handed** or **left-handed** surgeon. Both right and left hand tying will be demonstrated and illustrated and seen on CD ROM Disc 1. The most common types of two-hand ties are the square knot and the surgeon's knot. The knot is considered completed after 3 to 6 throws, depending on the material used and on the surgeon's preference. For instance, silk suture holds a knot well with 3 to 4 throws, while Prolene® suture is only secure after 5 to 7 throws. The CD-ROM on this subject will be very useful for learning the actual techniques of knot tying for both right - handed and left-handed surgeons. We will go through the steps of learning the two-hand tie (square knot and surgeon's knot) with illustrations and a piece of string. You can use an armchair and string to learn these knots **(Figure H-17)**. **Figures H-18, H-19** and **H-20** show how to make a square knot and surgeon's knot for the right handed surgeon. Instrument tie for right handed surgeon is on page 84, **Figure H-21**. All the ties for left handed surgeon begins on page 94, **Figure H-22, H-23, H-24 and H-25**.

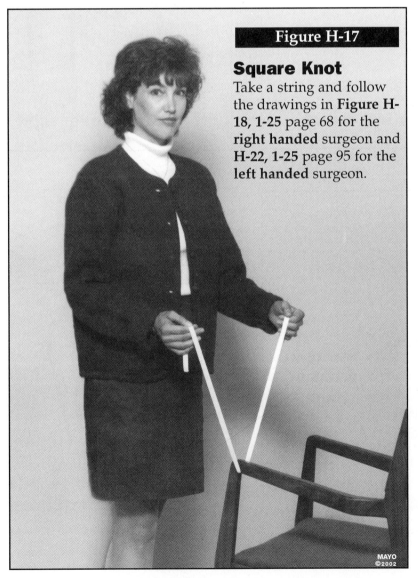

Figure H-17

Square Knot
Take a string and follow the drawings in **Figure H-18, 1-25** page 68 for the **right handed** surgeon and **H-22, 1-25** page 95 for the **left handed** surgeon.

MAYO
©2002

H. Sutures, Needles and Knots

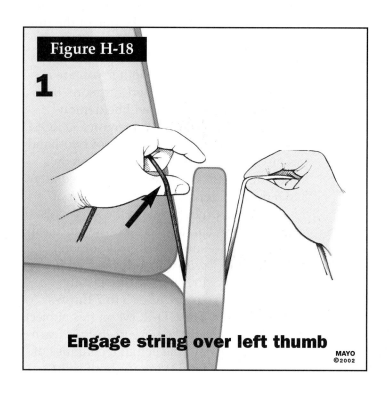

Figure H-18

1

Engage string over left thumb

MAYO
©2002

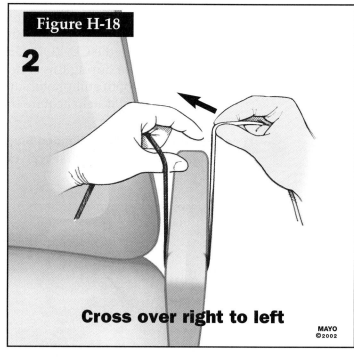

Figure H-18

2

Cross over right to left

MAYO
©2002

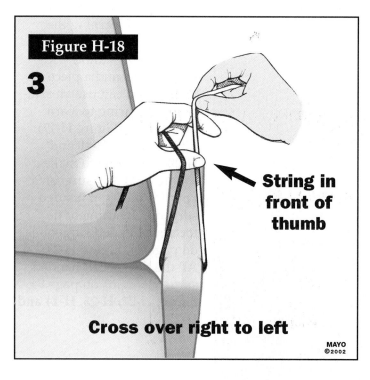

Figure H-18

3

String in front of thumb

Cross over right to left

MAYO
©2002

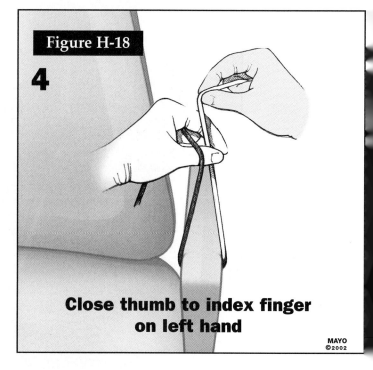

Figure H-18

4

Close thumb to index finger on left hand

MAYO
©2002

H. Sutures, Needles and Knots

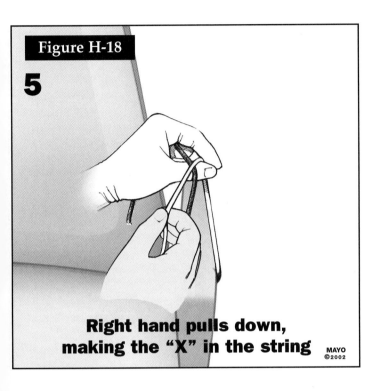

Figure H-18

5

Right hand pulls down, making the "X" in the string

MAYO ©2002

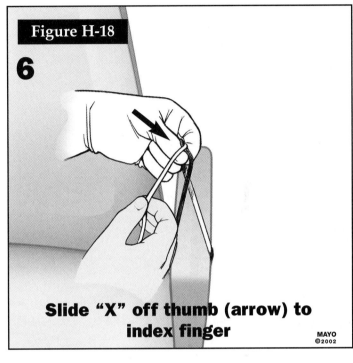

Figure H-18

6

Slide "X" off thumb (arrow) to index finger

MAYO ©2002

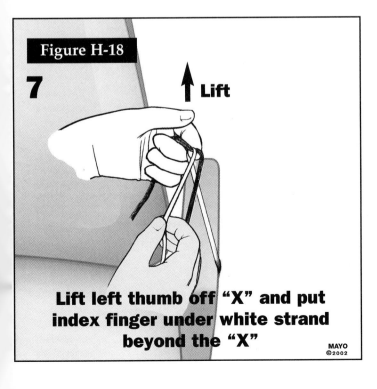

Figure H-18

7

↑ **Lift**

Lift left thumb off "X" and put index finger under white strand beyond the "X"

MAYO ©2002

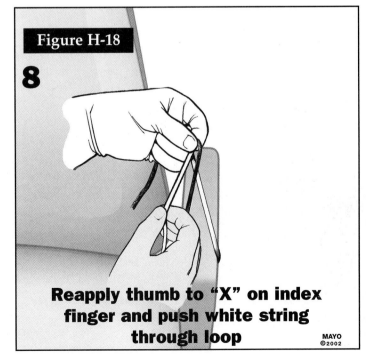

Figure H-18

8

Reapply thumb to "X" on index finger and push white string through loop

MAYO ©2002

69

H. Sutures, Needles and Knots

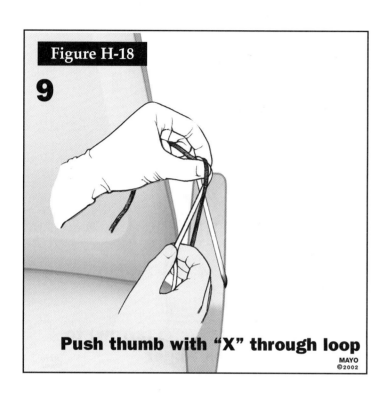

Figure H-18

9

Push thumb with "X" through loop

MAYO
©2002

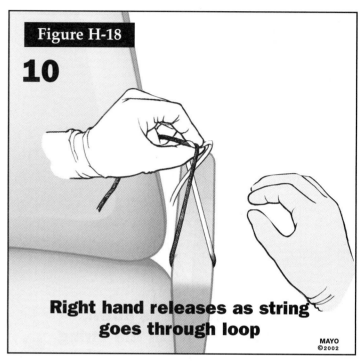

Figure H-18

10

Right hand releases as string
goes through loop

MAYO
©2002

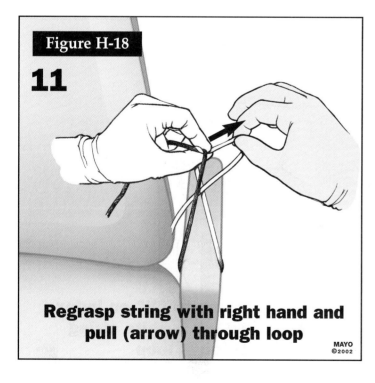

Figure H-18

11

Regrasp string with right hand and
pull (arrow) through loop

MAYO
©2002

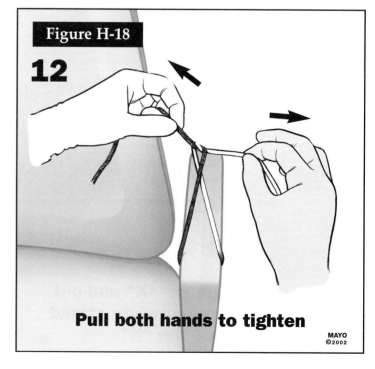

Figure H-18

12

Pull both hands to tighten

MAYO
©2002

H. Sutures, Needles and Knots

Figure H-18

13

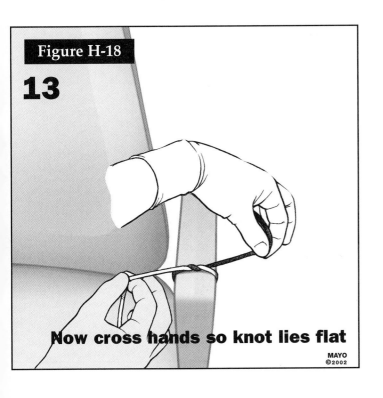

Now cross hands so knot lies flat

MAYO
©2002

Figure H-18

14

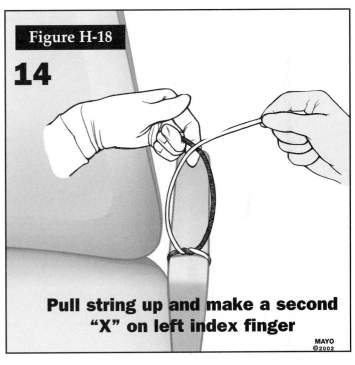

Pull string up and make a second "X" on left index finger

MAYO
©2002

Figure H-18

15

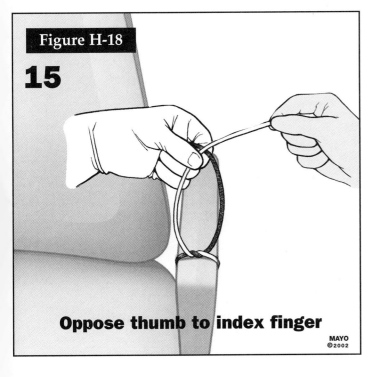

Oppose thumb to index finger

MAYO
©2002

Figure H-18

16

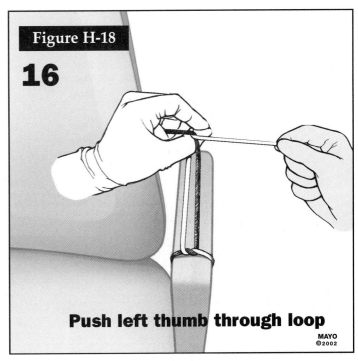

Push left thumb through loop

MAYO
©2002

H. Sutures, Needles and Knots

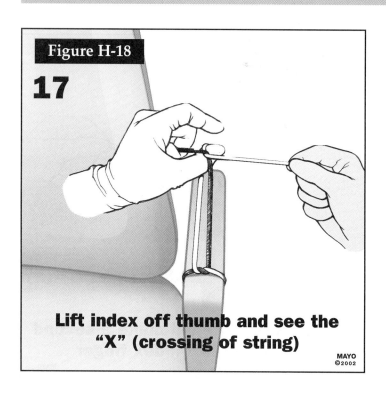

Figure H-18

17

Lift index off thumb and see the "X" (crossing of string)

MAYO ©2002

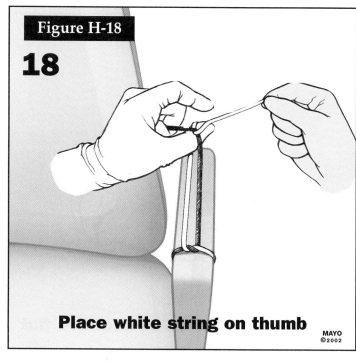

Figure H-18

18

Place white string on thumb

MAYO ©2002

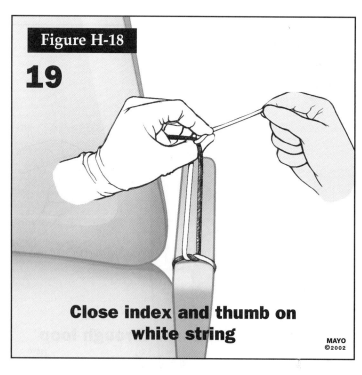

Figure H-18

19

Close index and thumb on white string

MAYO ©2002

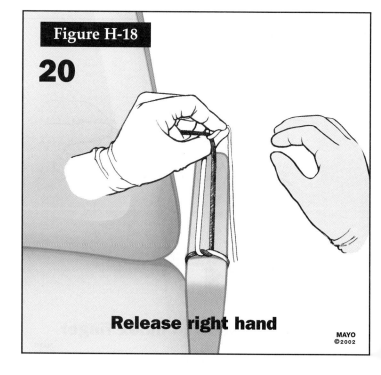

Figure H-18

20

Release right hand

MAYO ©2002

H. Sutures, Needles and Knots

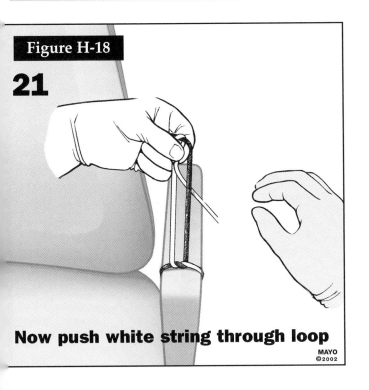

Figure H-18

21

Now push white string through loop

MAYO
©2002

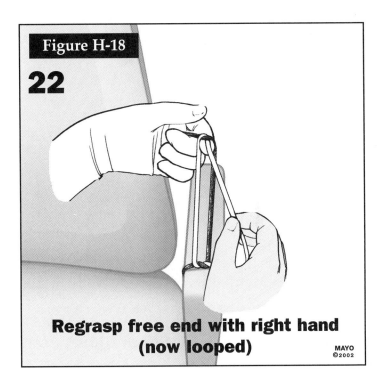

Figure H-18

22

Regrasp free end with right hand (now looped)

MAYO
©2002

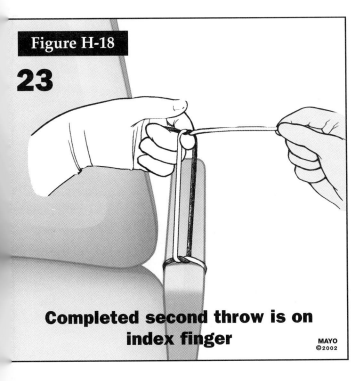

Figure H-18

23

Completed second throw is on index finger

MAYO
©2002

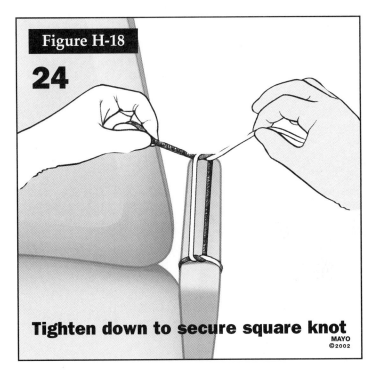

Figure H-18

24

Tighten down to secure square knot

MAYO
©2002

H. Sutures, Needles and Knots

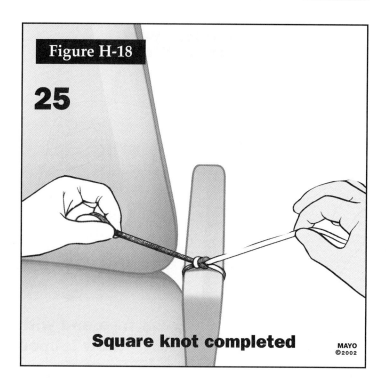

Figure H-18

25

Square knot completed

MAYO
©2002

Each twist a looping of suture to produce a knot is
called a throw. Most often 4 to 6 throws are placed
before a surgeon considers a knot completed. This is
to ensure that the knot is secure.

H. Sutures, Needles and Knots

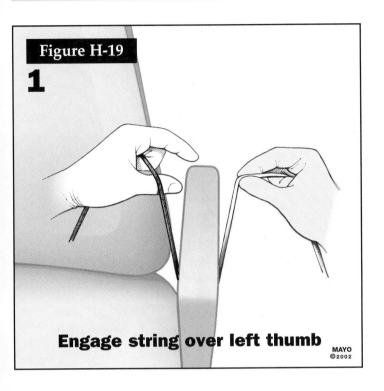

Figure H-19

1

Engage string over left thumb

MAYO
©2002

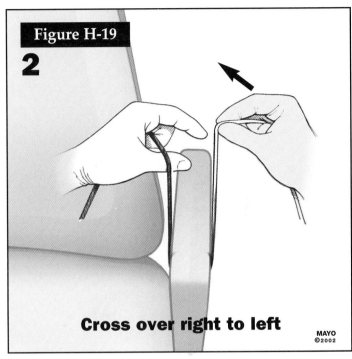

Figure H-19

2

Cross over right to left

MAYO
©2002

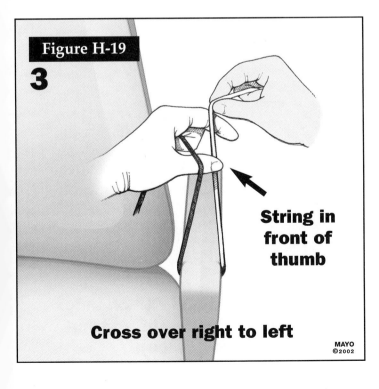

Figure H-19

3

String in front of thumb

Cross over right to left

MAYO
©2002

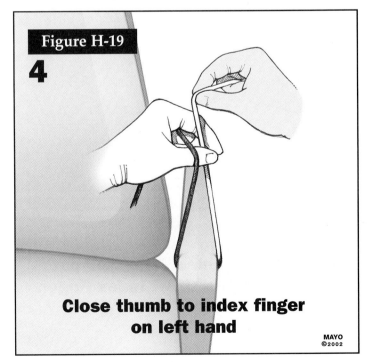

Figure H-19

4

Close thumb to index finger on left hand

MAYO
©2002

H. Sutures, Needles and Knots

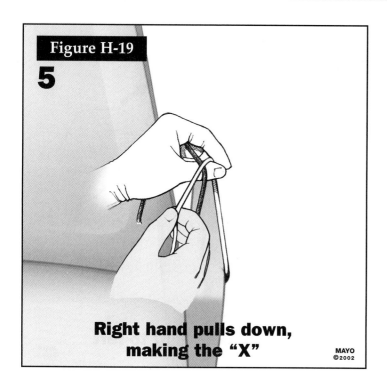

Figure H-19

5

Right hand pulls down, making the "X"

MAYO
©2002

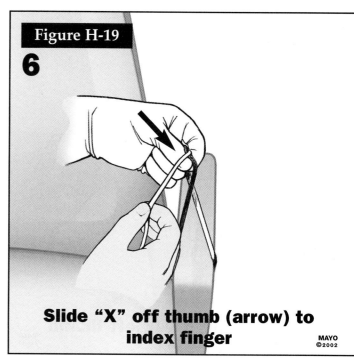

Figure H-19

6

Slide "X" off thumb (arrow) to index finger

MAYO
©2002

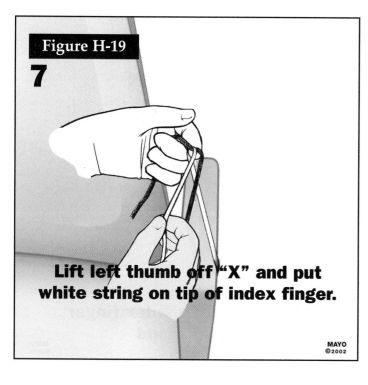

Figure H-19

7

Lift left thumb off "X" and put white string on tip of index finger.

MAYO
©2002

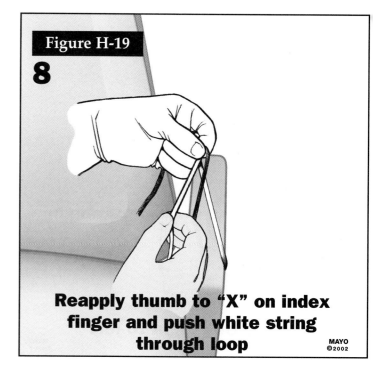

Figure H-19

8

Reapply thumb to "X" on index finger and push white string through loop

MAYO
©2002

H. Sutures, Needles and Knots

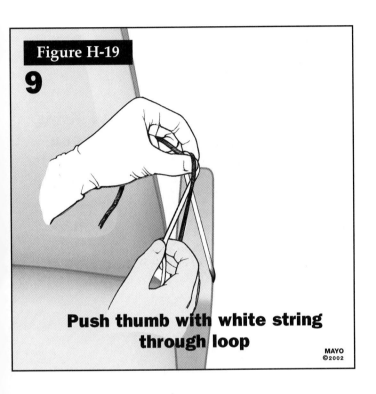

Figure H-19

9

Push thumb with white string through loop

MAYO
©2002

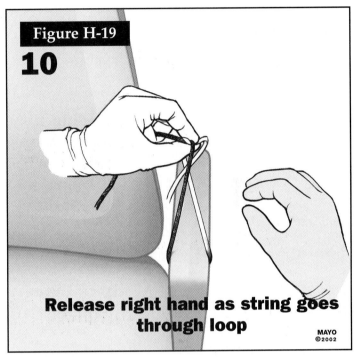

Figure H-19

10

Release right hand as string goes through loop

MAYO
©2002

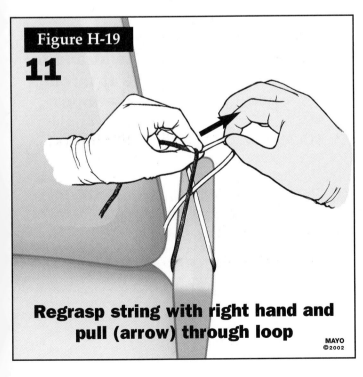

Figure H-19

11

Regrasp string with right hand and pull (arrow) through loop

MAYO
©2002

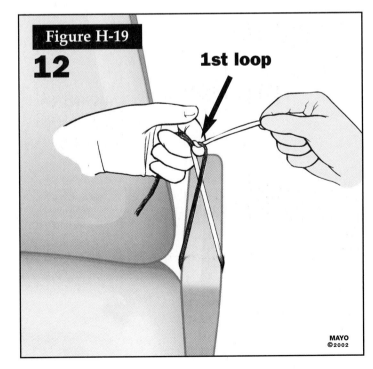

Figure H-19

12

1st loop

MAYO
©2002

H. Sutures, Needles and Knots

Figure H-19

13

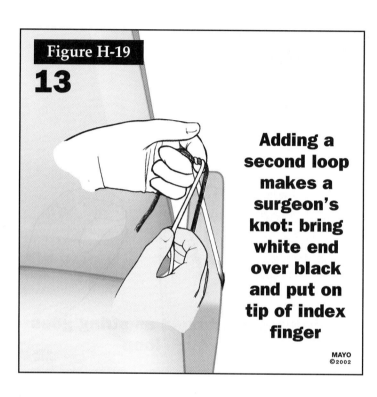

Adding a second loop makes a surgeon's knot: bring white end over black and put on tip of index finger

MAYO
©2002

Figure H-19

14

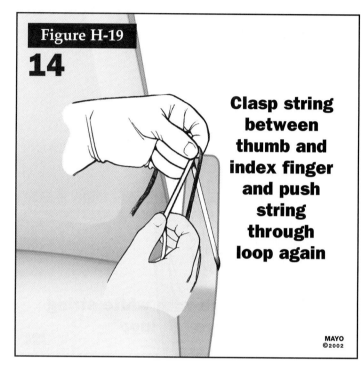

Clasp string between thumb and index finger and push string through loop again

MAYO
©2002

Figure H-19

15

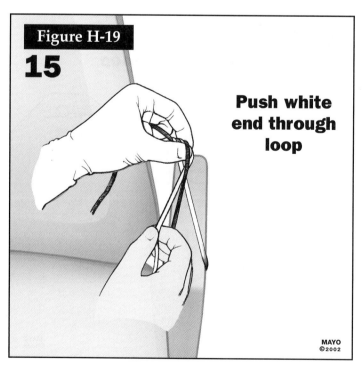

Push white end through loop

MAYO
©2002

Figure H-19

16

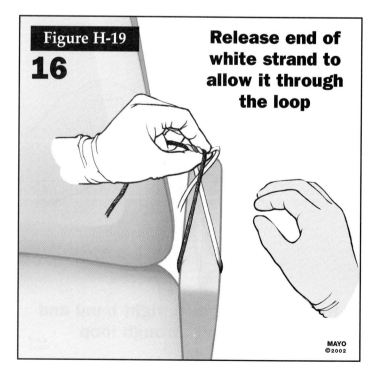

Release end of white strand to allow it through the loop

MAYO
©2002

H. Sutures, Needles and Knots

Figure H-19
17

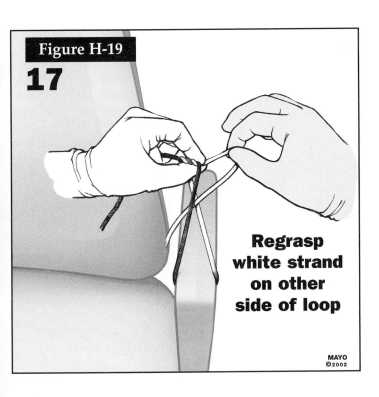

Regrasp white strand on other side of loop

MAYO
©2002

Figure H-19
18

2 loops

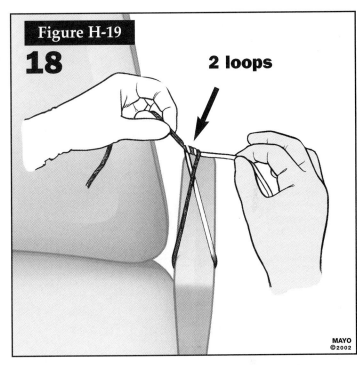

MAYO
©2002

Figure H-19
19

Pull down the double looped throw while crossing hands so that it is square

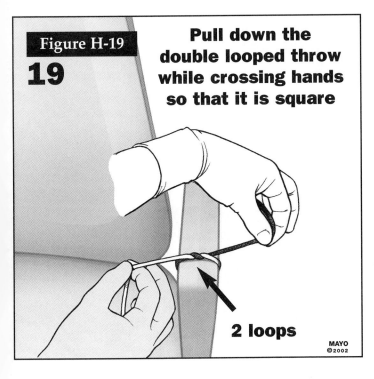

2 loops

MAYO
©2002

Figure H-19
20

Start next single loop

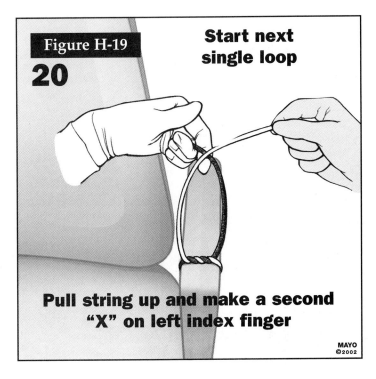

Pull string up and make a second "X" on left index finger

MAYO
©2002

H. Sutures, Needles and Knots

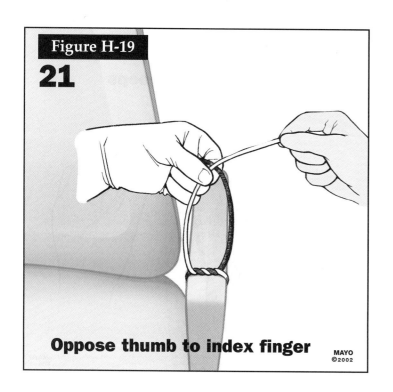

Figure H-19
21

Oppose thumb to index finger

MAYO ©2002

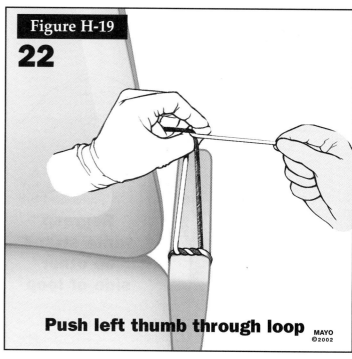

Figure H-19
22

Push left thumb through loop

MAYO ©2002

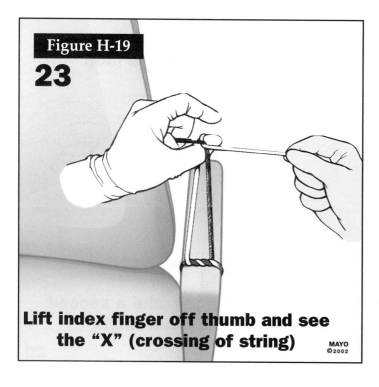

Figure H-19
23

Lift index finger off thumb and see the "X" (crossing of string)

MAYO ©2002

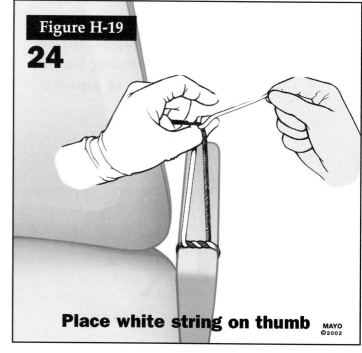

Figure H-19
24

Place white string on thumb

MAYO ©2002

H. Sutures, Needles and Knots

Figure H-19
25

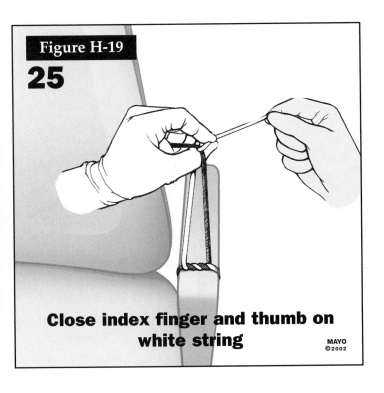

Close index finger and thumb on white string

MAYO
©2002

Figure H-19
26

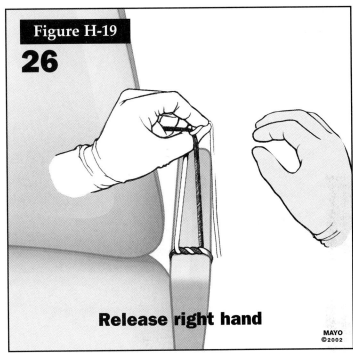

Release right hand

MAYO
©2002

Figure H-19
27

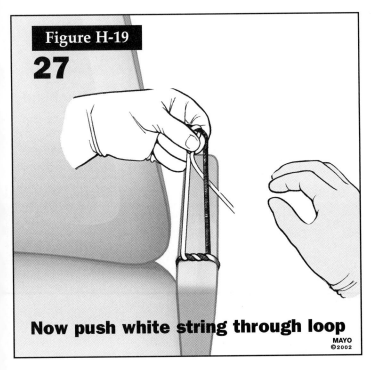

Now push white string through loop

MAYO
©2002

Figure H-19
28

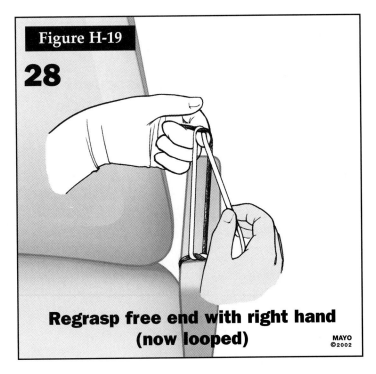

Regrasp free end with right hand (now looped)

MAYO
©2002

H. Sutures, Needles and Knots

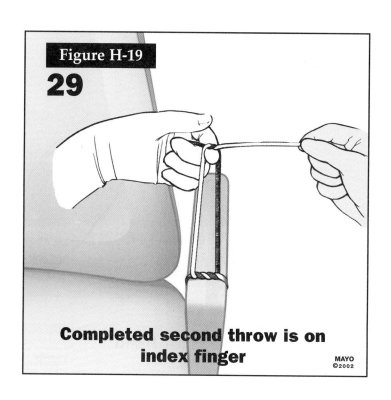

Figure H-19

29

Completed second throw is on index finger

MAYO
©2002

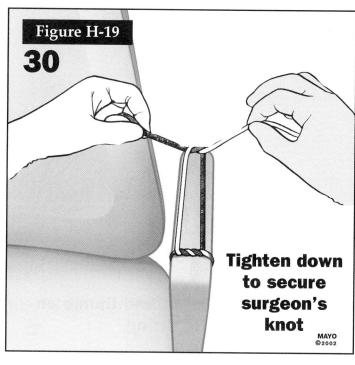

Figure H-19

30

Tighten down to secure surgeon's knot

MAYO
©2002

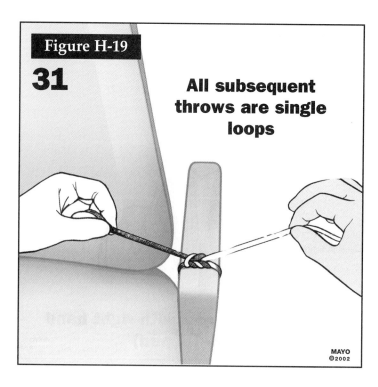

Figure H-19

31

All subsequent throws are single loops

MAYO
©2002

Comparison Between Square Knot and Surgeon's Knot

The square knot has one loop in the first throw, while the the surgeon's knot has two loops **(Figure H-20,1,2).** After the first throw is completed the rest of the tie is the same in both knots. Subsequent throws are always opposite the previous throw to improve the security of the tie. When practicing knot tying, do as many throws as the string allows to make the hand motions second nature. The surgeon's knot is useful because the first throw with the two loops **(Figure H-20, 2)** tends to stay in place better than the square knot with its one loop prior to place-ment of the second throw. **Figure H-20, 3-4** shows the square knot and surgeon's knot secure.

H. Sutures, Needles and Knots

TWO-HAND TIE — COMPARISON BETWEEN SURGEON'S AND SQUARE KNOT — RIGHT HANDED SURGEON

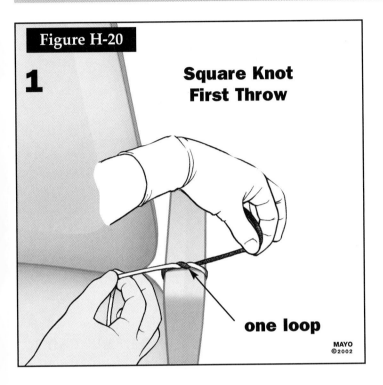

Figure H-20

1

Square Knot First Throw

one loop

MAYO
©2002

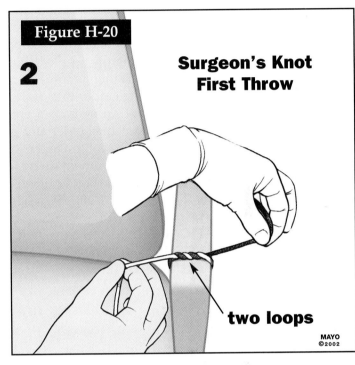

Figure H-20

2

Surgeon's Knot First Throw

two loops

MAYO
©2002

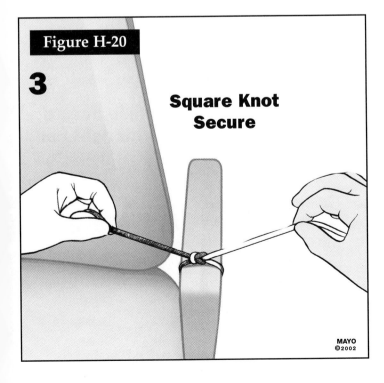

Figure H-20

3

Square Knot Secure

MAYO
©2002

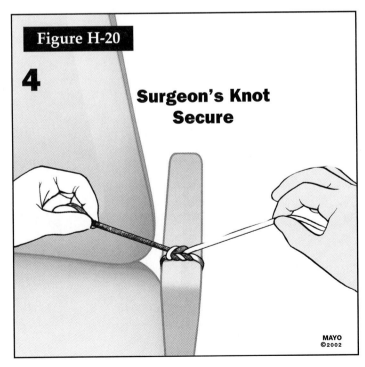

Figure H-20

4

Surgeon's Knot Secure

MAYO
©2002

H. Sutures, Needles and Knots

b. Instrument Tie - Right Handed Surgeon

The instrument tie is extremely useful and has a variety of applications, especially in facial surgery. Surgeon's knots and square knots are also used with the instrument tie. In this tie, the needle holder is kept in one hand after passing the needle through the tissue. The suture is then wrapped around the end of the needle holder to make a loop. The short, free end of suture is then grasped in the jaws of the needle holder and pulled through the loop to complete the knot. You can practice the instrument tie by using a silk suture (2-0), a needle holder (driver), and a towel **(Figure H-21: 1-20)**. Two-hand ties can also be practiced with this suture. **IT IS CRITICAL THAT YOU MASTER BOTH THE TWO HAND TIE AND THE INSTRUMENT TIE.**

INSTRUMENT TIE WITH SURGEON'S KNOT — RIGHT HANDED SURGEON

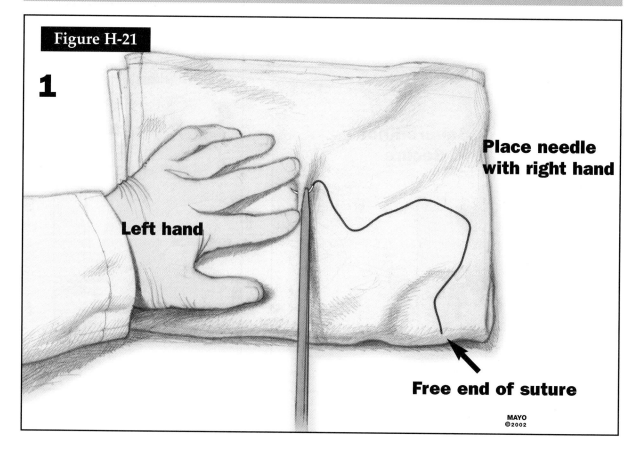

Figure H-21

1

Place needle with right hand

Left hand

Free end of suture

MAYO
©2002

H. Sutures, Needles and Knots

Figure H-21

2

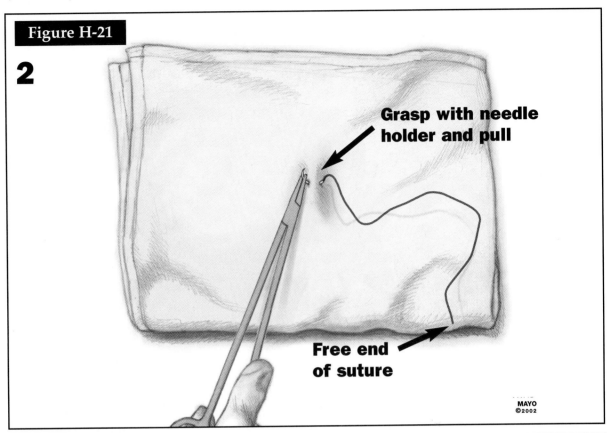

Grasp with needle holder and pull

Free end of suture

MAYO
©2002

Figure H-21

3

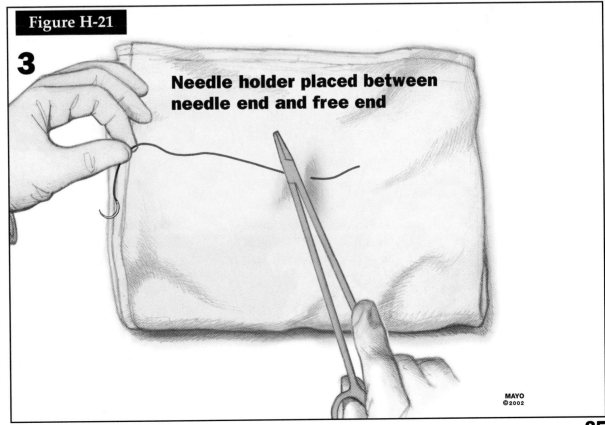

Needle holder placed between needle end and free end

MAYO
©2002

H. Sutures, Needles and Knots

Figure H-21

4

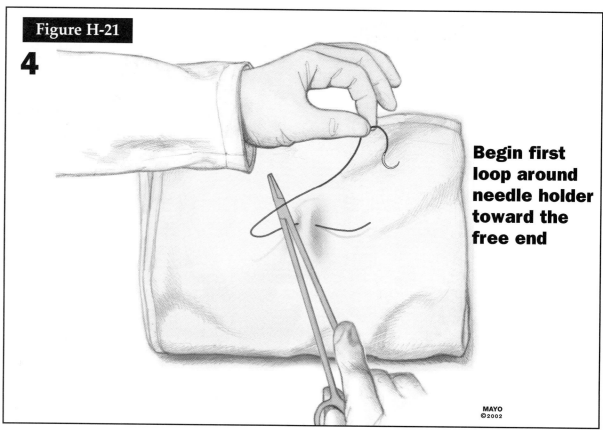

Begin first loop around needle holder toward the free end

MAYO
©2002

Figure H-21

5

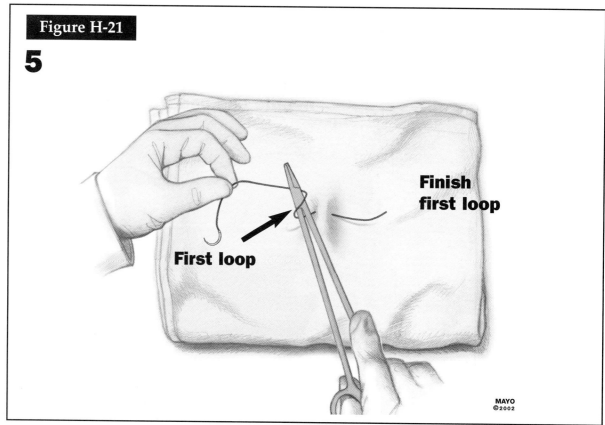

Finish first loop

First loop

MAYO
©2002

H. Sutures, Needles and Knots

Figure H-21

6

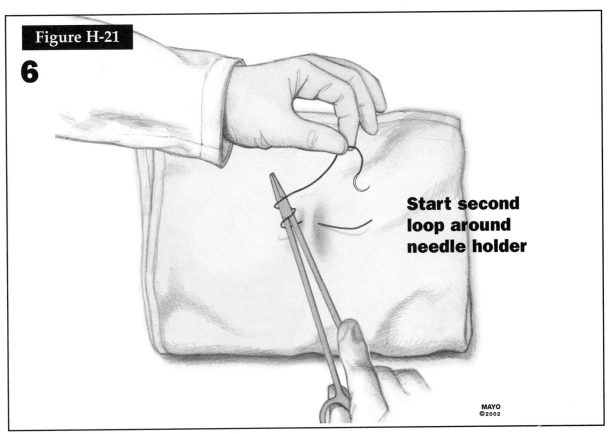

Start second loop around needle holder

MAYO
©2002

Figure H-21

7

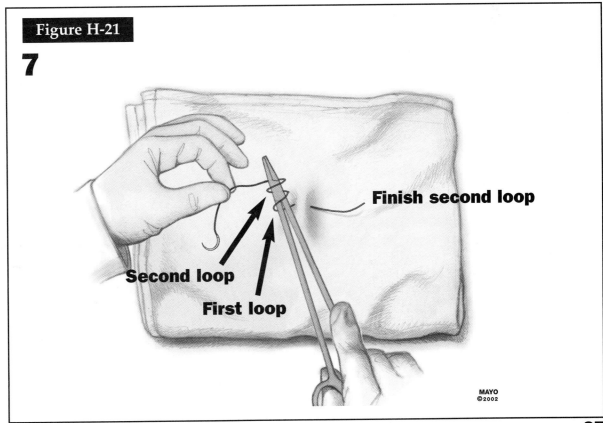

Finish second loop

Second loop

First loop

MAYO
©2002

H. Sutures, Needles and Knots

Figure H-21

8

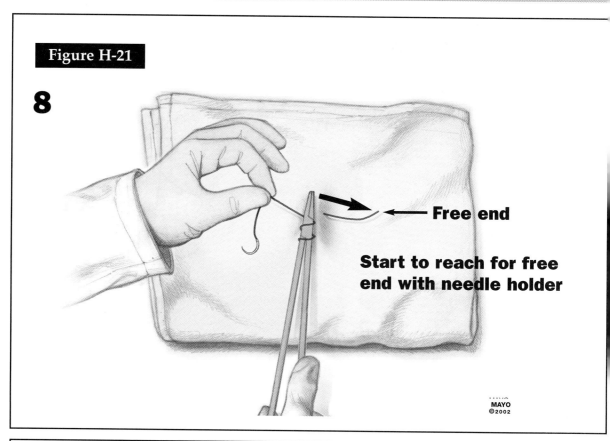

← **Free end**

Start to reach for free end with needle holder

MAYO
©2002

Figure H-21

9

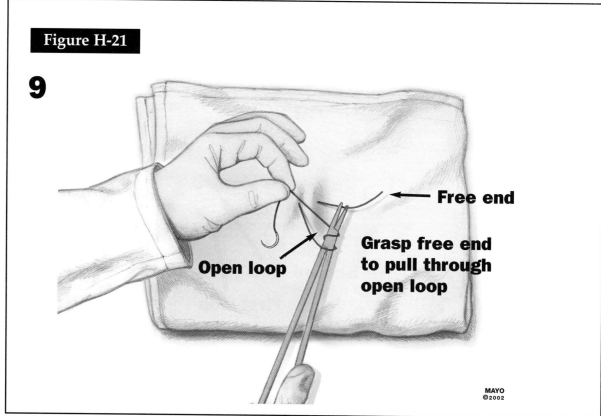

← **Free end**

Open loop

Grasp free end to pull through open loop

MAYO
©2002

H. Sutures, Needles and Knots

Figure H-21

10

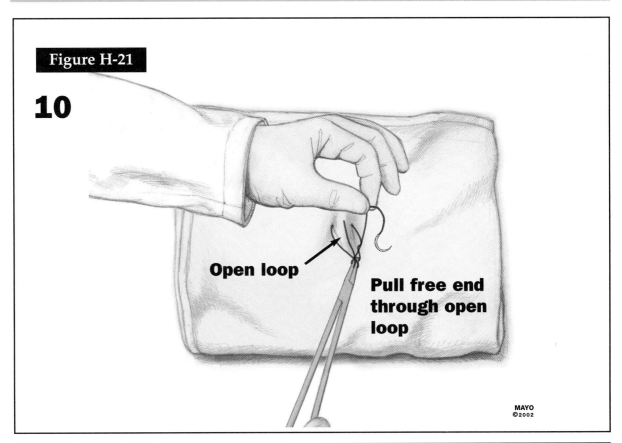

Open loop

Pull free end through open loop

MAYO
©2002

Figure H-21

11

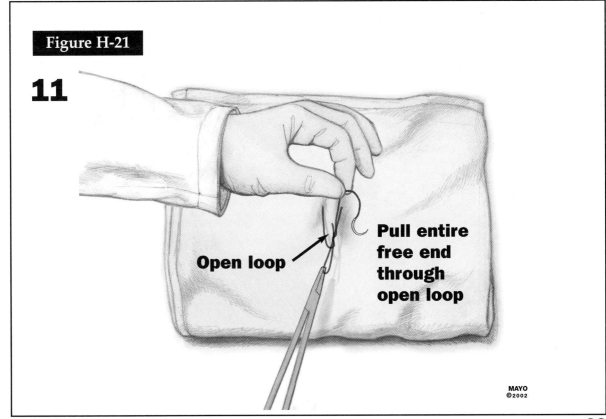

Open loop

Pull entire free end through open loop

MAYO
©2002

H. Sutures, Needles and Knots

Figure H-21

12

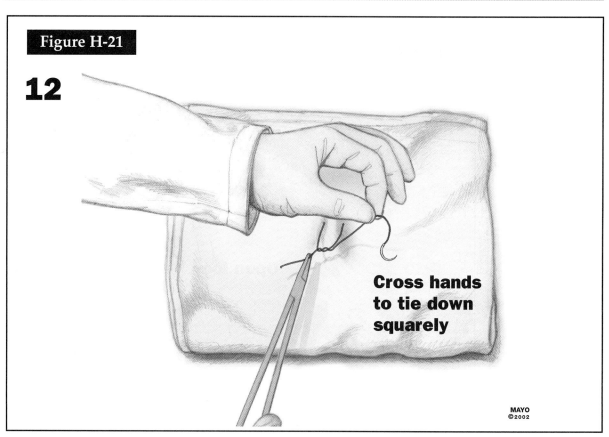

**Cross hands
to tie down
squarely**

MAYO
©2002

Figure H-21

13

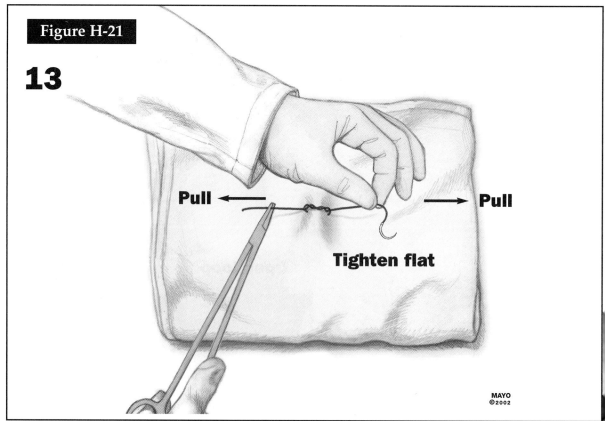

Pull ←   → **Pull**

Tighten flat

MAYO
©2002

H. Sutures, Needles and Knots

Figure H-21

14

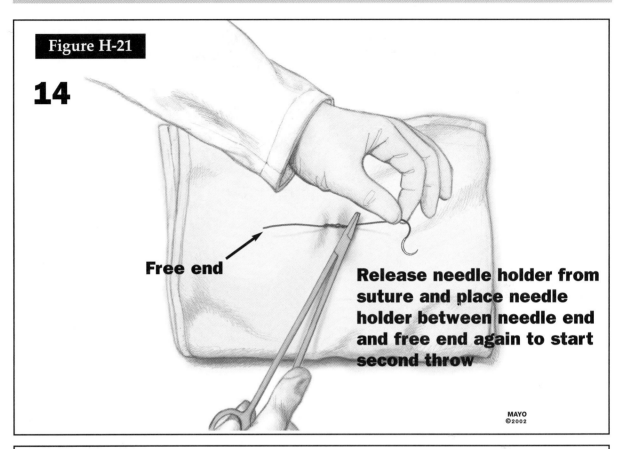

Free end

Release needle holder from suture and place needle holder between needle end and free end again to start second throw

MAYO
©2002

Figure H-21

15

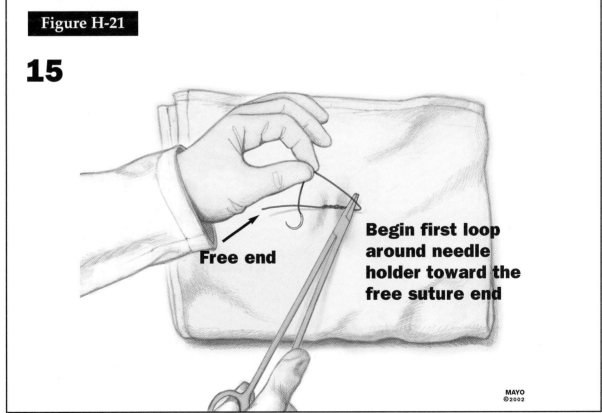

Free end

Begin first loop around needle holder toward the free suture end

MAYO
©2002

H. Sutures, Needles and Knots

Figure H-21

16

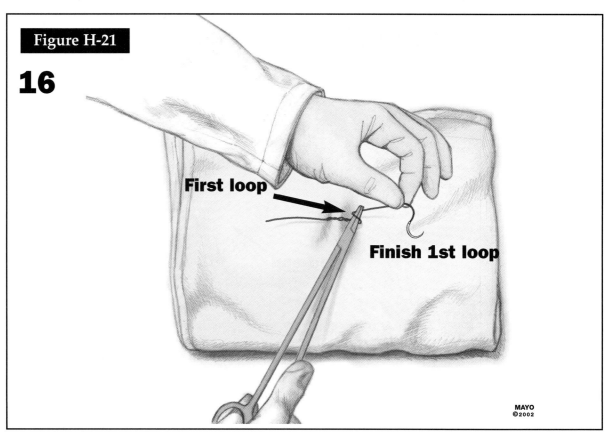

First loop

Finish 1st loop

MAYO
©2002

Figure H-21

17

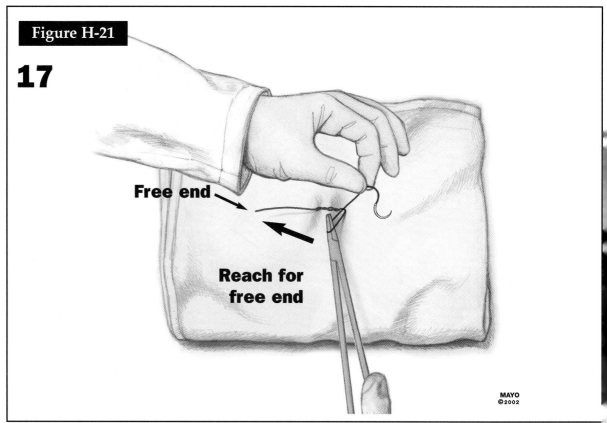

Free end

Reach for
free end

MAYO
©2002

H. Sutures, Needles and Knots

Figure H-21

18

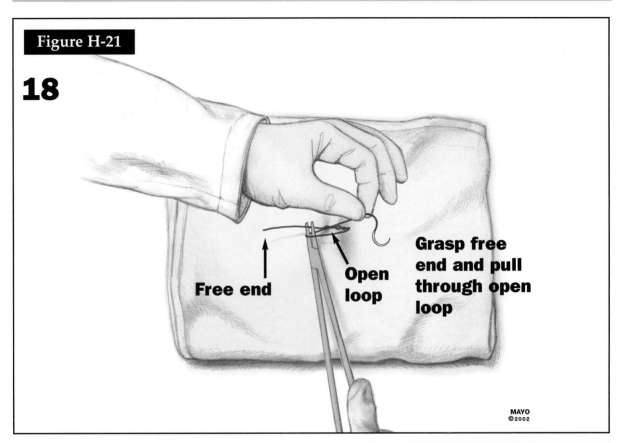

Free end

Open loop

Grasp free end and pull through open loop

MAYO
©2002

Figure H-21

19

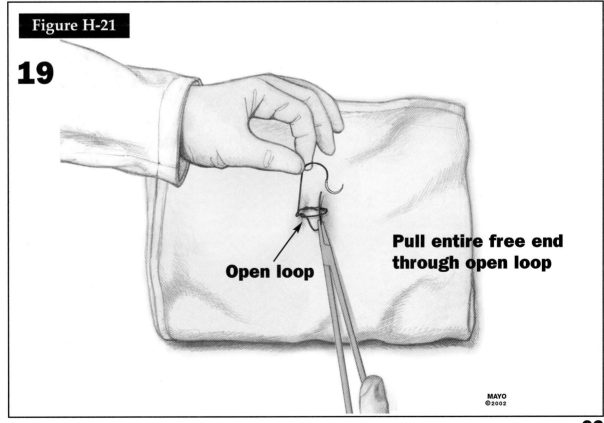

Open loop

Pull entire free end through open loop

MAYO
©2002

H. Sutures, Needles and Knots

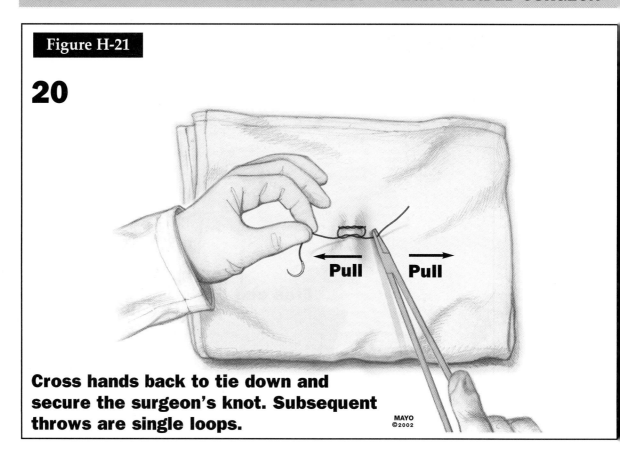

Figure H-21

20

Cross hands back to tie down and secure the surgeon's knot. Subsequent throws are single loops.

MAYO ©2002

c. Two-Hand Tie - Left Handed Surgeon
Figure **H-22, 1-25** demonstrates two-handed tie square knot. **Figure H-23, 1-31** demonstrates two-hand tie surgeon's knot for the left handed surgeon.

H. Sutures, Needles and Knots

Figure H-22

1

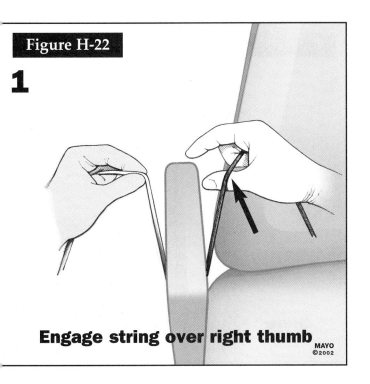

Engage string over right thumb MAYO ©2002

Figure H-22

2

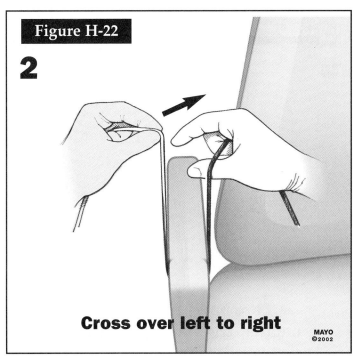

Cross over left to right MAYO ©2002

Figure H-22

3

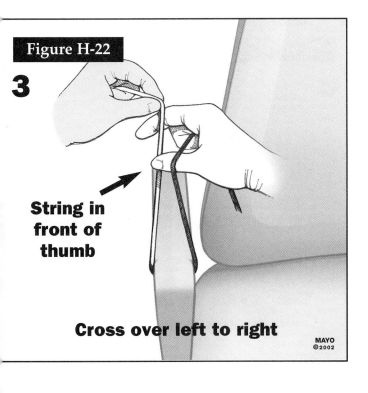

String in front of thumb

Cross over left to right MAYO ©2002

Figure H-22

4

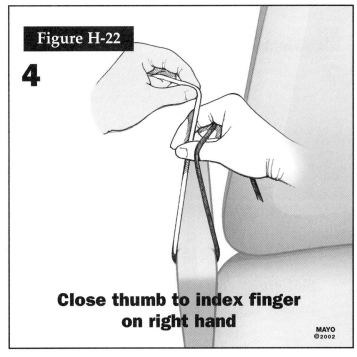

Close thumb to index finger on right hand MAYO ©2002

H. Sutures, Needles and Knots

Figure H-22

5

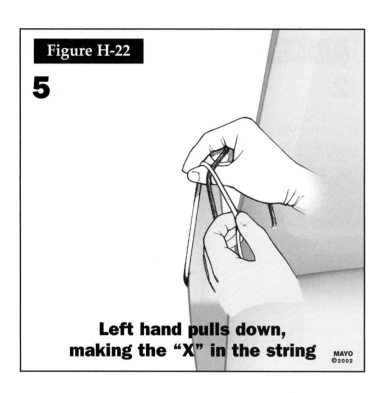

Left hand pulls down, making the "X" in the string

MAYO
©2002

Figure H-22

6

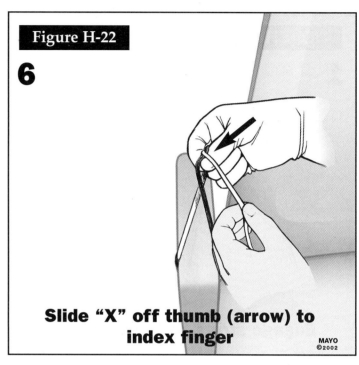

Slide "X" off thumb (arrow) to index finger

MAYO
©2002

Figure H-22

7

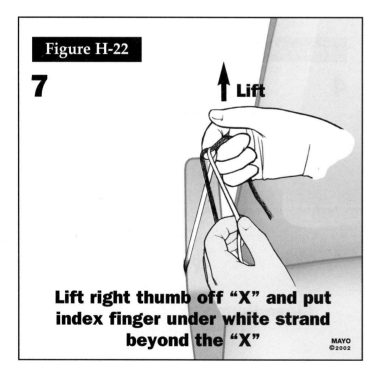

↑ Lift

Lift right thumb off "X" and put index finger under white strand beyond the "X"

MAYO
©2002

Figure H-22

8

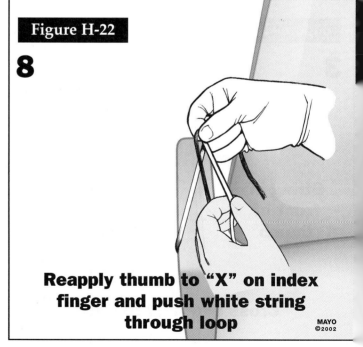

Reapply thumb to "X" on index finger and push white string through loop

MAYO
©2002

H. Sutures, Needles and Knots

TWO-HAND TIE — SQUARE KNOT — LEFT HANDED SURGEON

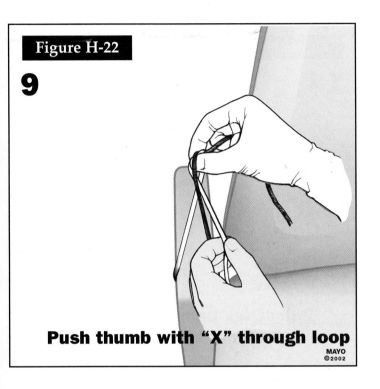

Figure H-22

9

Push thumb with "X" through loop

MAYO
©2002

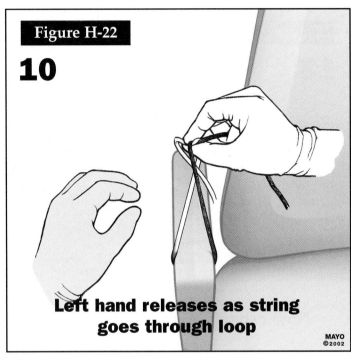

Figure H-22

10

Left hand releases as string
goes through loop

MAYO
©2002

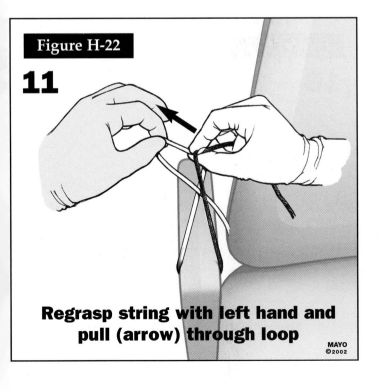

Figure H-22

11

Regrasp string with left hand and
pull (arrow) through loop

MAYO
©2002

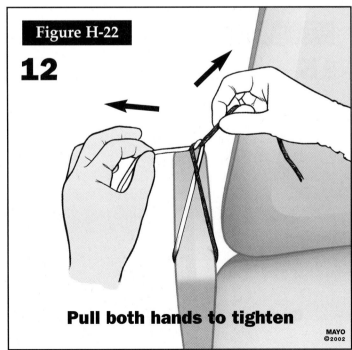

Figure H-22

12

Pull both hands to tighten

MAYO
©2002

H. Sutures, Needles and Knots

Figure H-22

13

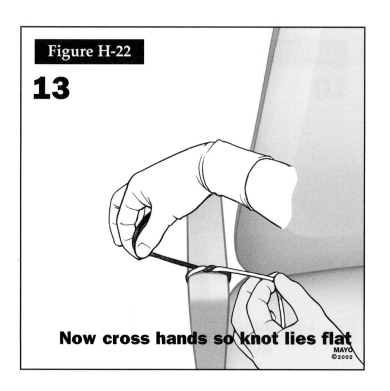

Now cross hands so knot lies flat

MAYO
©2002

Figure H-22

14

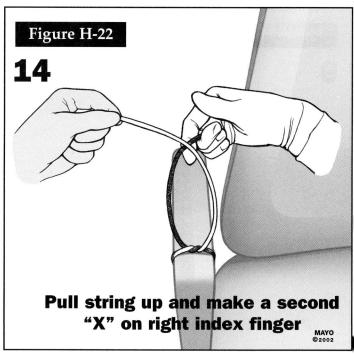

Pull string up and make a second "X" on right index finger

MAYO
©2002

Figure H-22

15

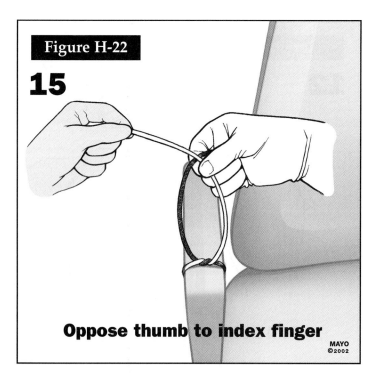

Oppose thumb to index finger

MAYO
©2002

Figure H-22

16

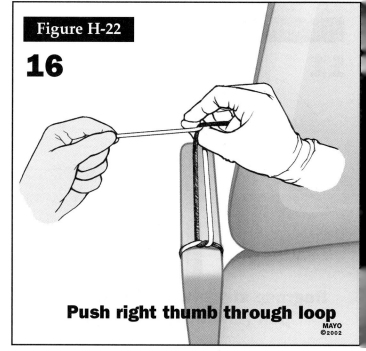

Push right thumb through loop

MAYO
©2002

H. Sutures, Needles and Knots

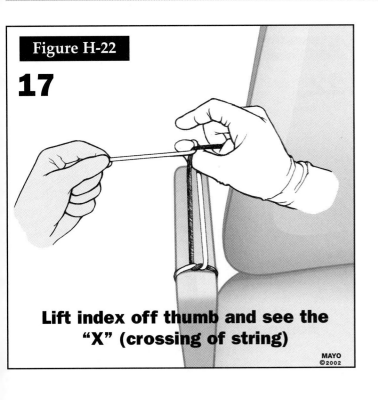

Figure H-22

17

Lift index off thumb and see the "X" (crossing of string)

MAYO
©2002

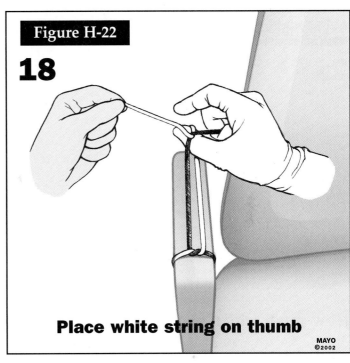

Figure H-22

18

Place white string on thumb

MAYO
©2002

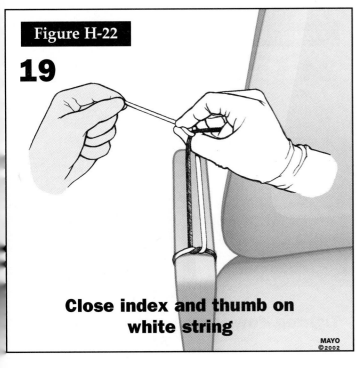

Figure H-22

19

Close index and thumb on white string

MAYO
©2002

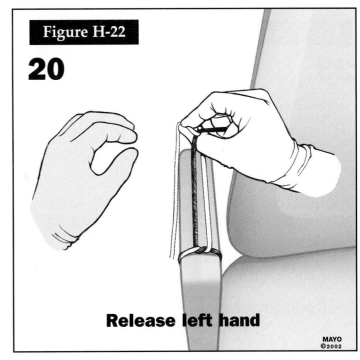

Figure H-22

20

Release left hand

MAYO
©2002

H. Sutures, Needles and Knots

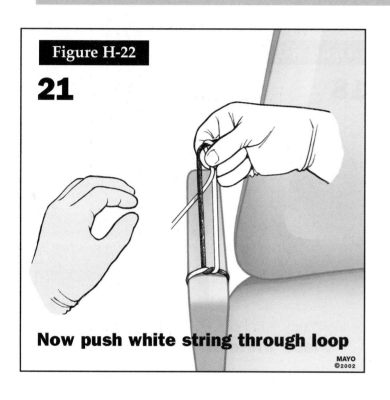

Figure H-22

21

Now push white string through loop

MAYO
©2002

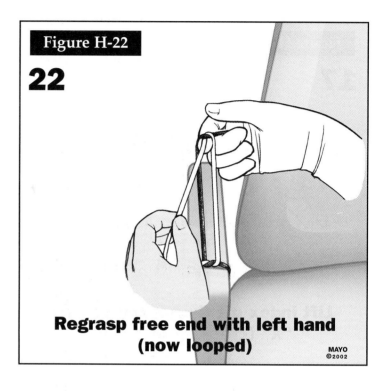

Figure H-22

22

Regrasp free end with left hand (now looped)

MAYO
©2002

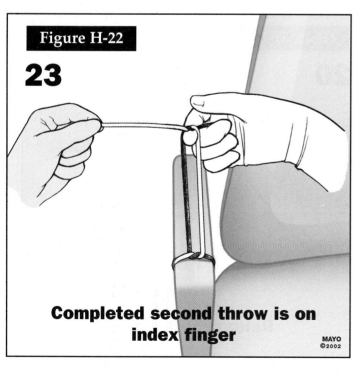

Figure H-22

23

Completed second throw is on index finger

MAYO
©2002

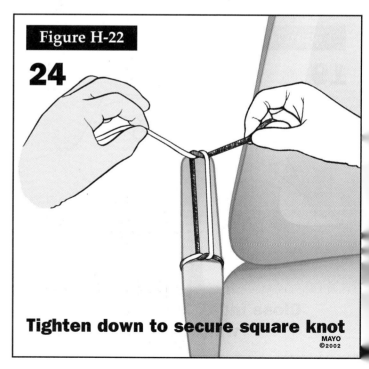

Figure H-22

24

Tighten down to secure square knot

MAYO
©2002

H. Sutures, Needles and Knots

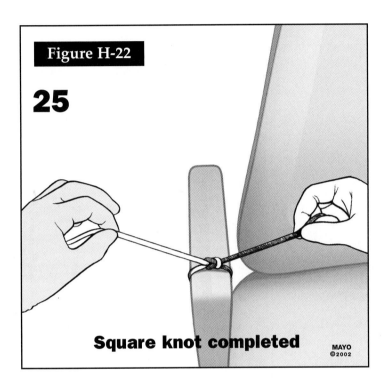

Figure H-22

25

Square knot completed

MAYO
©2002

Most often 4 to 6 throws are placed before a surgeon considers a knot completed. This is to ensure the security of the knot.

H. Sutures, Needles and Knots

TWO-HAND TIE — SURGEON'S KNOT — LEFT HANDED SURGEON

Figure **H-23, 1-31** demonstrates the two-hand tie surgeon's knot for the left handed surgeon.

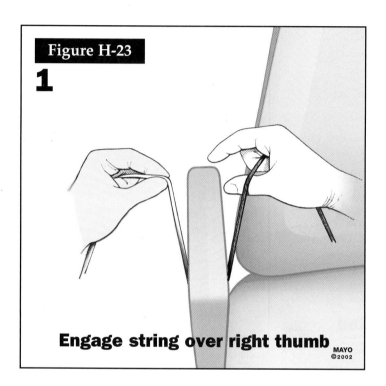

Figure H-23

1

Engage string over right thumb

MAYO
©2002

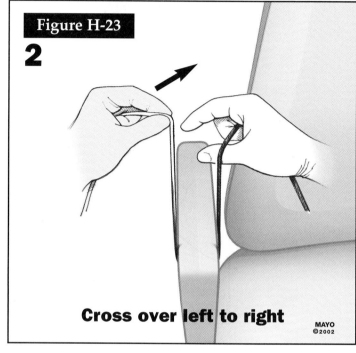

Figure H-23

2

Cross over left to right

MAYO
©2002

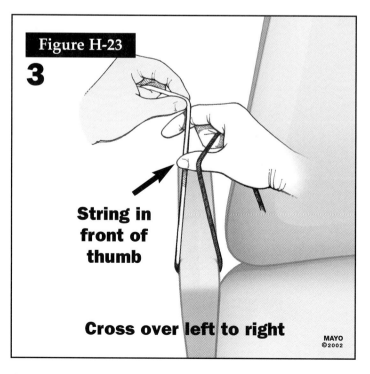

Figure H-23

3

String in front of thumb

Cross over left to right

MAYO
©2002

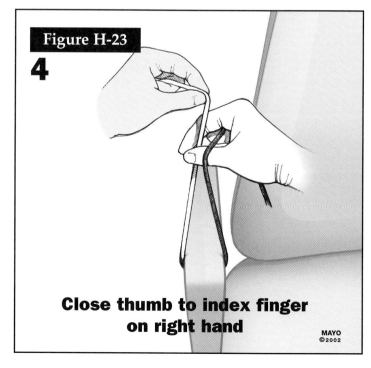

Figure H-23

4

Close thumb to index finger on right hand

MAYO
©2002

H. Sutures, Needles and Knots

Figure H-23

5

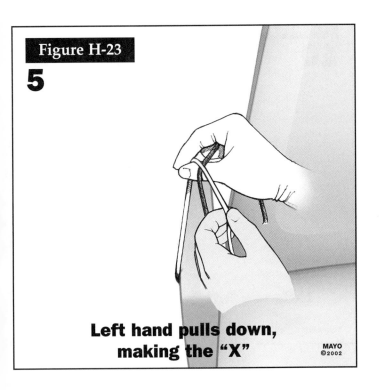

Left hand pulls down, making the "X"

MAYO
©2002

Figure H-23

6

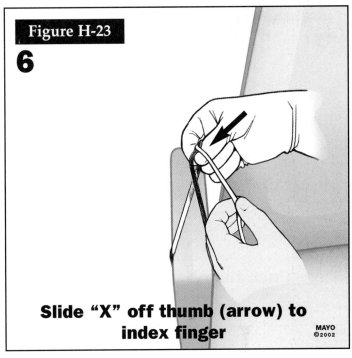

Slide "X" off thumb (arrow) to index finger

MAYO
©2002

Figure H-23

7

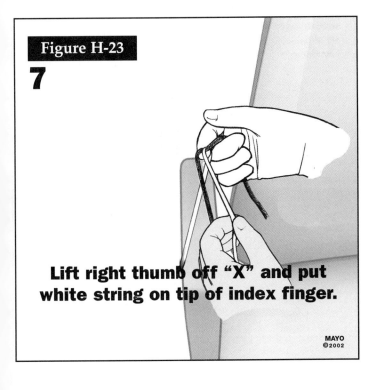

Lift right thumb off "X" and put white string on tip of index finger.

MAYO
©2002

Figure H-23

8

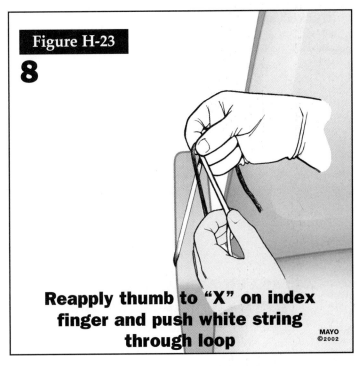

Reapply thumb to "X" on index finger and push white string through loop

MAYO
©2002

H. Sutures, Needles and Knots

Figure H-23

9

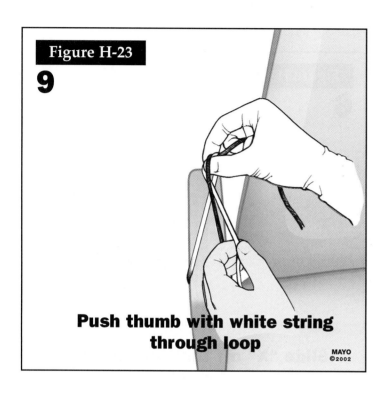

Push thumb with white string through loop

MAYO
©2002

Figure H-23

10

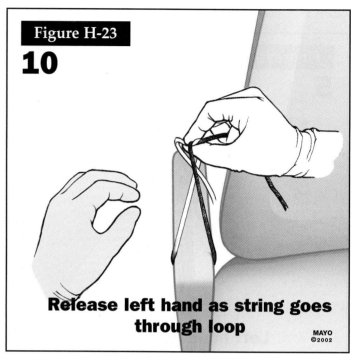

Release left hand as string goes through loop

MAYO
©2002

Figure H-23

11

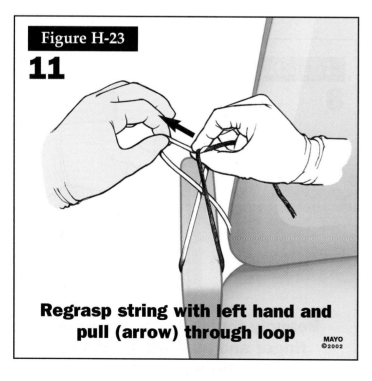

Regrasp string with left hand and pull (arrow) through loop

MAYO
©2002

Figure H-23

12   1st loop

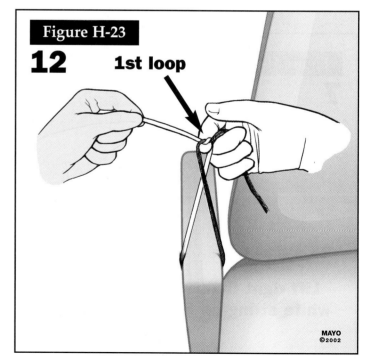

MAYO
©2002

H. Sutures, Needles and Knots

Figure H-23

13

Adding a second loop makes a surgeon's knot: bring white end over black and put on tip of index finger

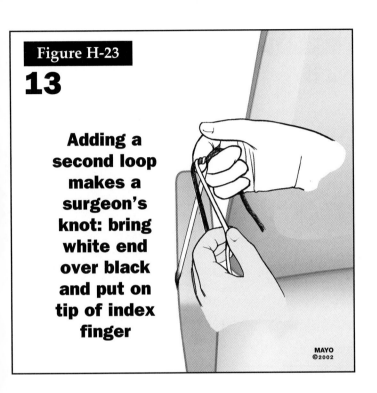

MAYO
©2002

Figure H-23

14

Clasp string between thumb and index finger and push string through loop again

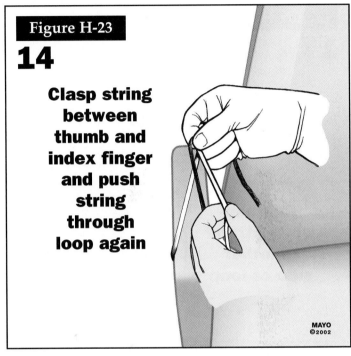

MAYO
©2002

Figure H-23

15

Push white end through loop

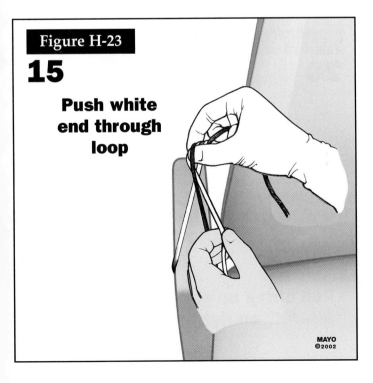

MAYO
©2002

Figure H-23

16

Release end of white strand to allow it through the loop

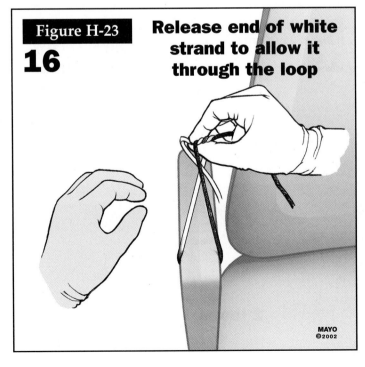

MAYO
©2002

H. Sutures, Needles and Knots

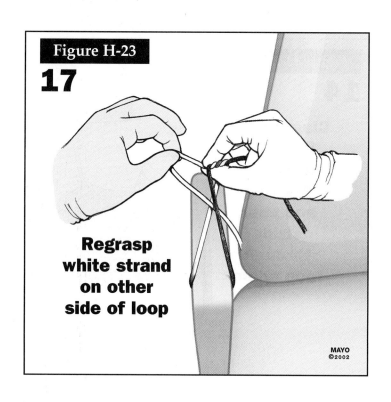

Figure H-23

17

Regrasp white strand on other side of loop

MAYO ©2002

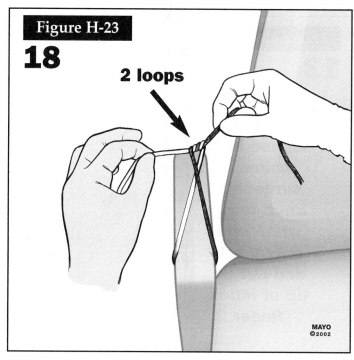

Figure H-23

18

2 loops

MAYO ©2002

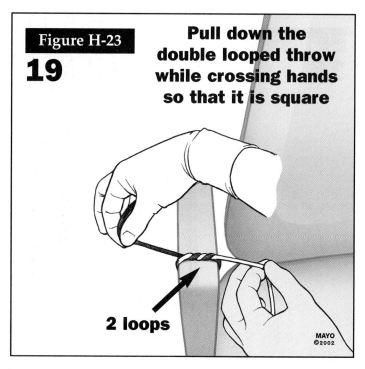

Figure H-23

19

Pull down the double looped throw while crossing hands so that it is square

2 loops

MAYO ©2002

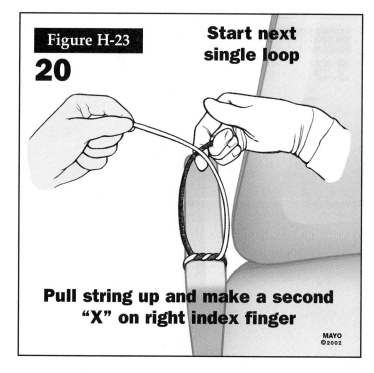

Figure H-23

20

Start next single loop

Pull string up and make a second "X" on right index finger

MAYO ©2002

H. Sutures, Needles and Knots

Figure H-23
21

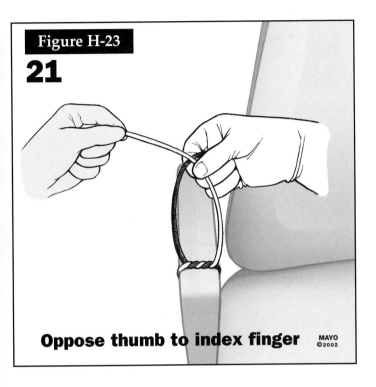

Oppose thumb to index finger MAYO ©2002

Figure H-23
22

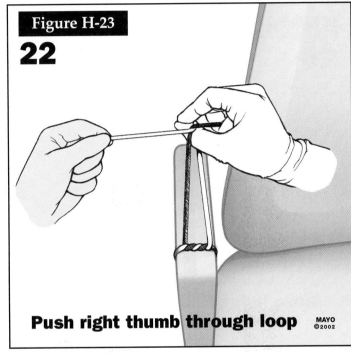

Push right thumb through loop MAYO ©2002

Figure H-23
23

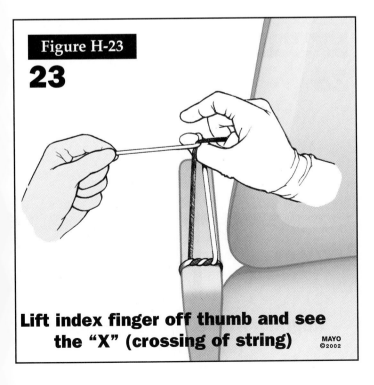

Lift index finger off thumb and see the "X" (crossing of string) MAYO ©2002

Figure H-23
24

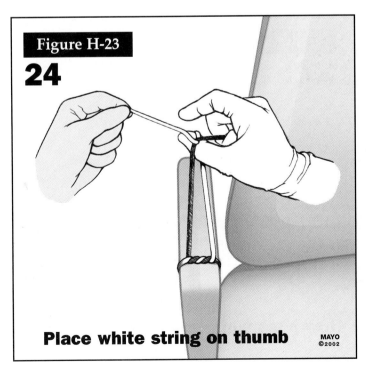

Place white string on thumb MAYO ©2002

107

H. Sutures, Needles and Knots

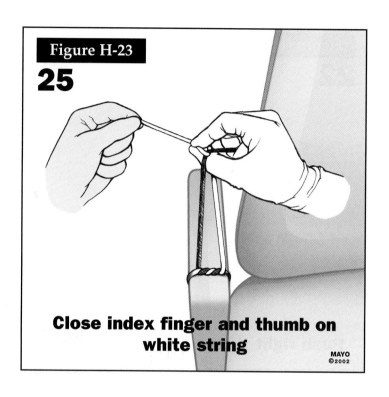

Figure H-23
25

Close index finger and thumb on white string

MAYO
©2002

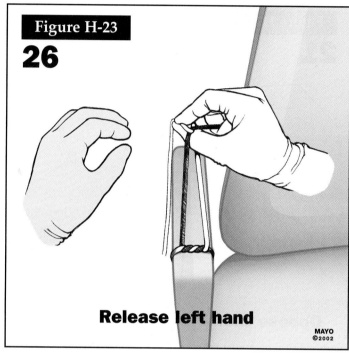

Figure H-23
26

Release left hand

MAYO
©2002

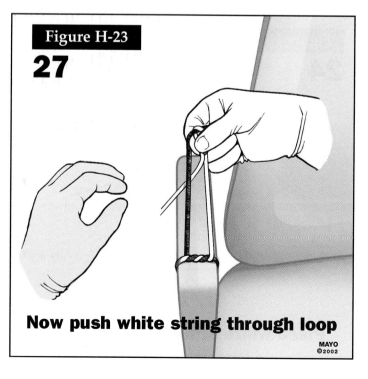

Figure H-23
27

Now push white string through loop

MAYO
©2002

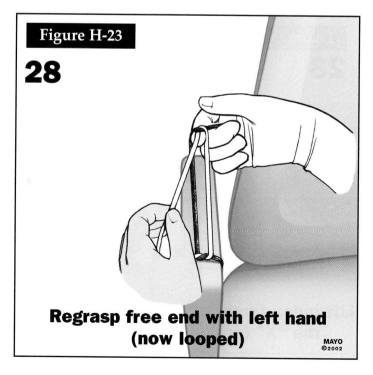

Figure H-23
28

Regrasp free end with left hand (now looped)

MAYO
©2002

H. Sutures, Needles and Knots

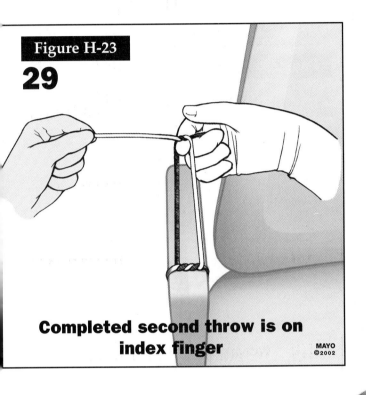

Figure H-23

29

Completed second throw is on index finger

MAYO ©2002

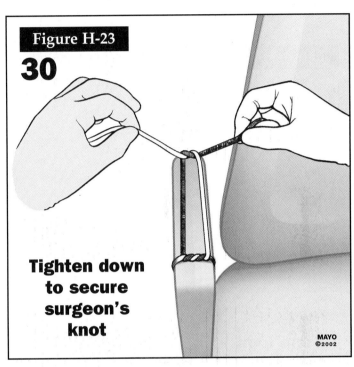

Figure H-23

30

Tighten down to secure surgeon's knot

MAYO ©2002

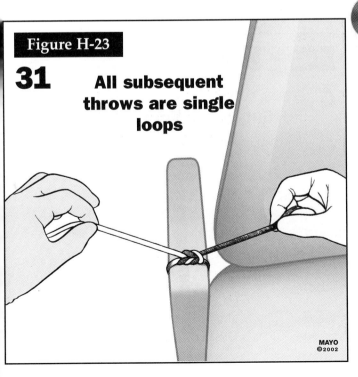

Figure H-23

31 **All subsequent throws are single loops**

MAYO ©2002

TWO-HAND TIE — COMPARISON BETWEEN SQUARE KNOT AND SURGEON'S KNOT

Comparison Between Square Knot and Surgeon's Knot

If you did not understand the difference between the square knot and the surgeon's knot, recheck **Figure H-24**, and read the text below.

The square knot has one loop in the first throw, while the the surgeon's knot has two loops **(Figure H-24:1,2)**. After the first throw is completed the rest of the tie is the same in both knots. Subsequent throws are always opposite the previous throw to improve the security of the tie. When practicing knot tying, do as many throws as the string allows to make the hand motions second nature. The surgeon's knot is useful because the first throw with the two loops **(Figure H-24:2)** tends to stay in place better than the square knot with its one loop prior to placement of the second throw. **Figure H-24: 3,4** shows the square knot and surgeon's knot secure.

109

H. Sutures, Needles and Knots

TWO-HAND TIE — COMPARISON BETWEEN SURGEON'S AND SQUARE KNOT — LEFT HANDED SURGEON

Figure H-24, 1-4 demonstrates the comparison between the surgeon's knot and the square knot for the left handed surgeon.

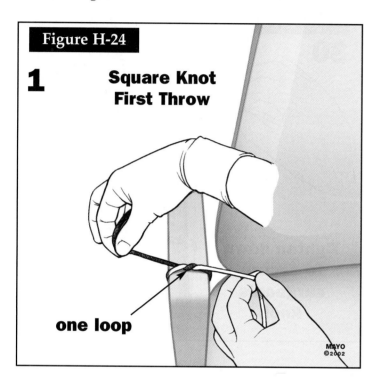

Figure H-24

1 **Square Knot First Throw**

one loop

MAYO
©2002

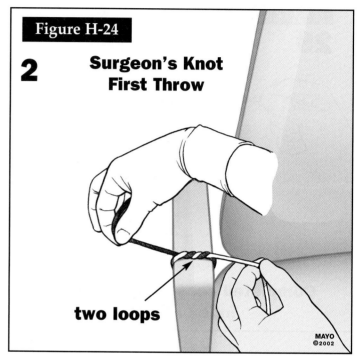

Figure H-24

2 **Surgeon's Knot First Throw**

two loops

MAYO
©2002

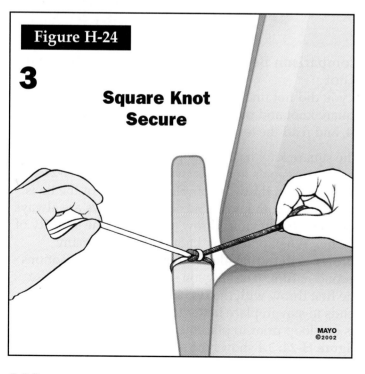

Figure H-24

3 **Square Knot Secure**

MAYO
©2002

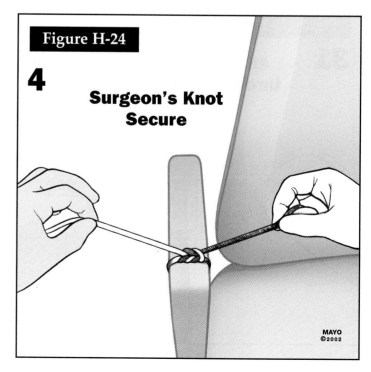

Figure H-24

4 **Surgeon's Knot Secure**

MAYO
©2002

H. Sutures, Needles and Knots

d. Instrument Tie - Left Handed Surgeon

Figure H-25, 1-20 demonstrates the instrument tie with surgeon's knot for the left handed surgeon.

INSTRUMENT TIE WITH SURGEON'S KNOT - LEFT HANDED SURGEON

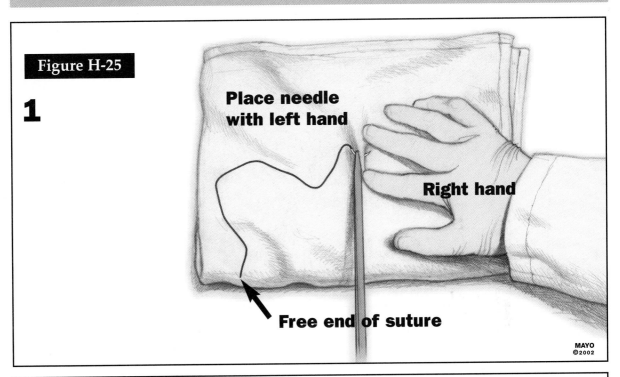

Figure H-25

1

Place needle with left hand

Right hand

Free end of suture

MAYO
©2002

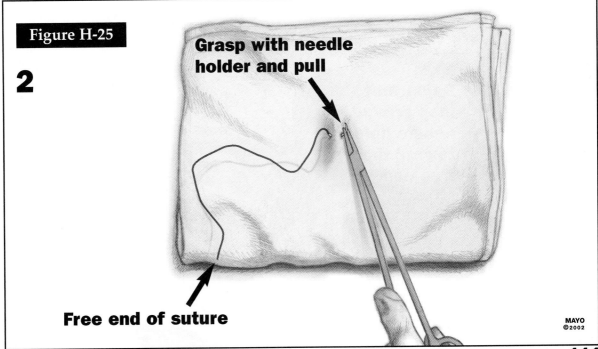

Figure H-25

2

Grasp with needle holder and pull

Free end of suture

MAYO
©2002

H. Sutures, Needles and Knots

INSTRUMENT TIE WITH SURGEON'S KNOT - LEFT HANDED SURGEON

Figure H-25

3

Needle holder place between needle end an free end

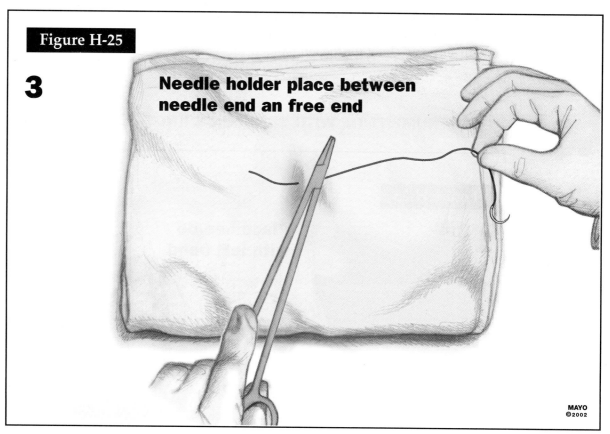

MAYO
©2002

Figure H-25

4

Begin first loop around needle holder toward the free end.

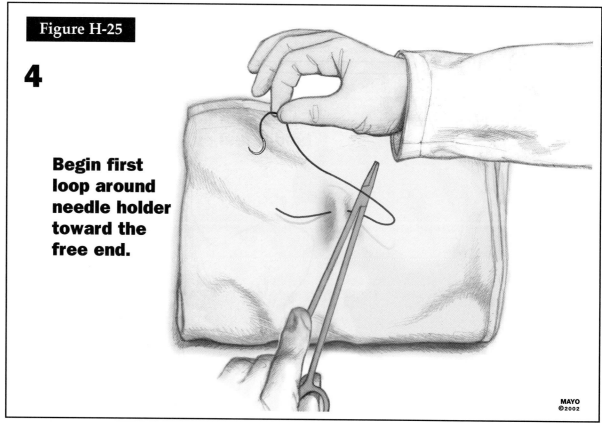

MAYO
©2002

H. Sutures, Needles and Knots

Figure H-25

5

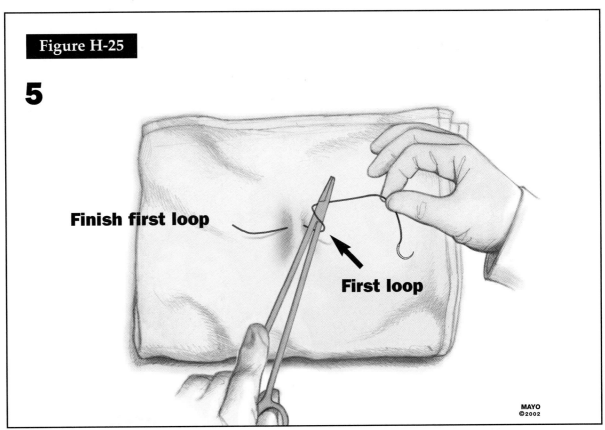

Finish first loop

First loop

MAYO
©2002

Figure H-25

6

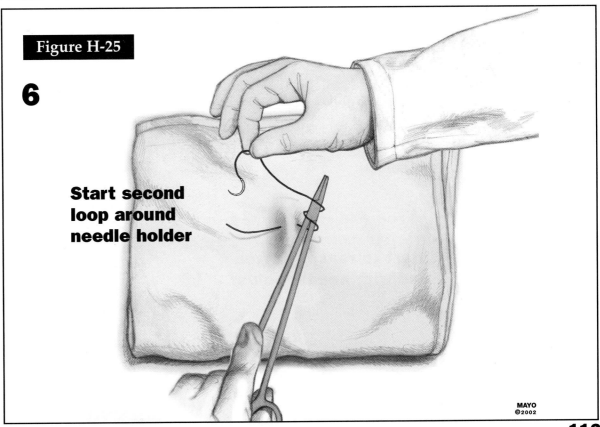

Start second loop around needle holder

MAYO
©2002

H. Sutures, Needles and Knots

Figure H-25

7

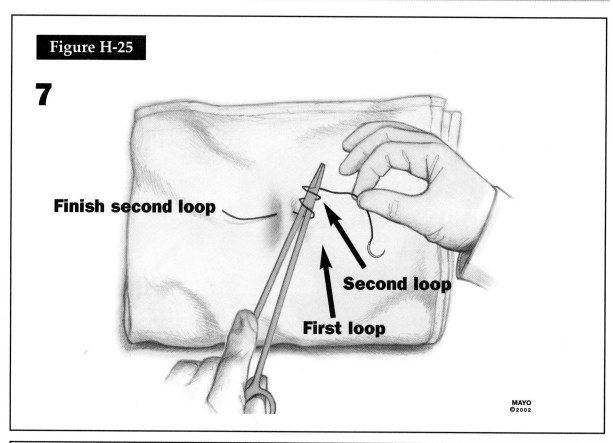

Finish second loop

Second loop

First loop

MAYO
©2002

Figure H-25

8

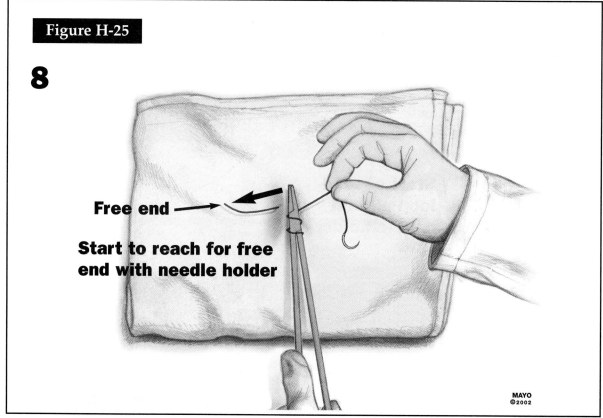

Free end

Start to reach for free
end with needle holder

MAYO
©2002

H. Sutures, Needles and Knots

Figure H-25

9

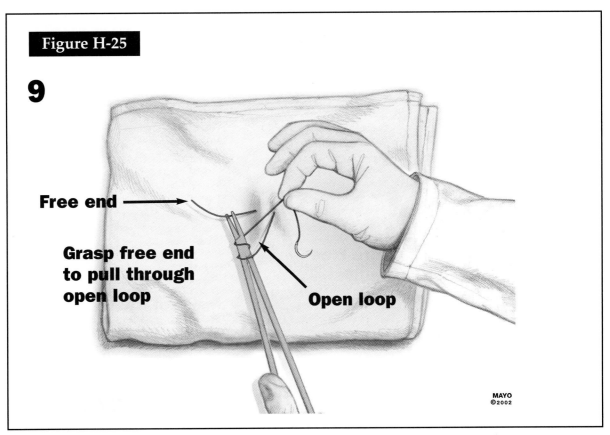

Free end

**Grasp free end
to pull through
open loop**

Open loop

MAYO
©2002

Figure H-25

10

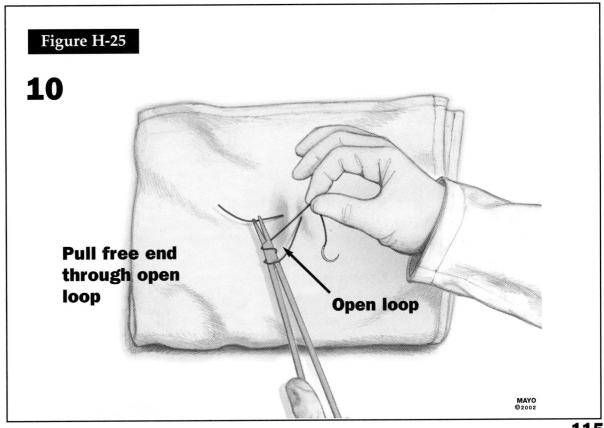

**Pull free end
through open
loop**

Open loop

MAYO
©2002

H. Sutures, Needles and Knots

Figure H-25

11

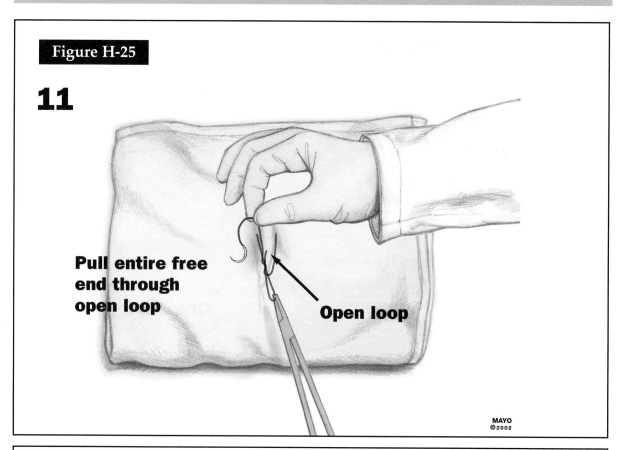

Pull entire free
end through
open loop

Open loop

MAYO
©2002

Figure H-25

12

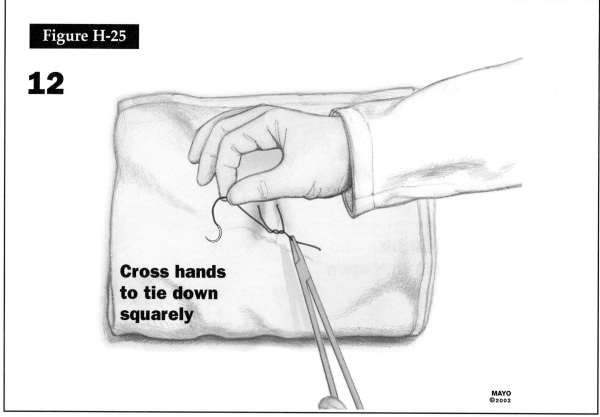

Cross hands
to tie down
squarely

MAYO
©2002

H. Sutures, Needles and Knots

INSTRUMENT TIE WITH SURGEON'S KNOT - LEFT HANDED SURGEON

Figure H-25

13

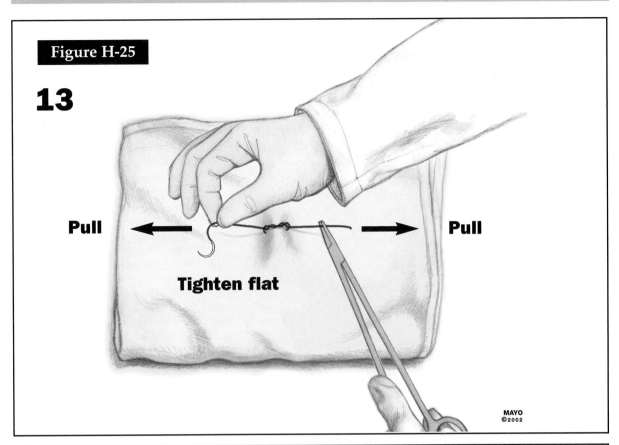

Pull ← → Pull

Tighten flat

MAYO
©2002

Figure H-25

14

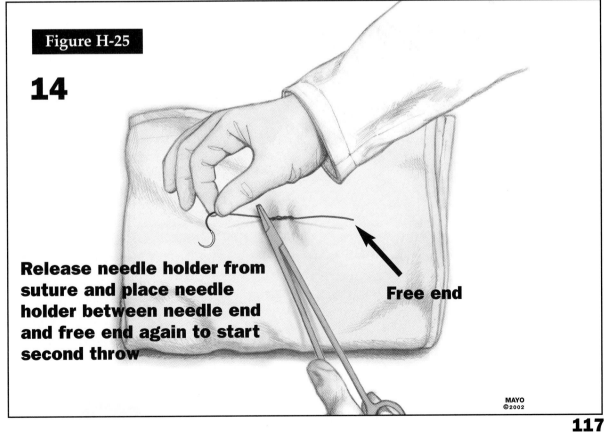

Release needle holder from suture and place needle holder between needle end and free end again to start second throw

Free end

MAYO
©2002

H. Sutures, Needles and Knots

INSTRUMENT TIE WITH SURGEON'S KNOT - LEFT HANDED SURGEON

15

Begin first loop around needle holder toward the free suture end

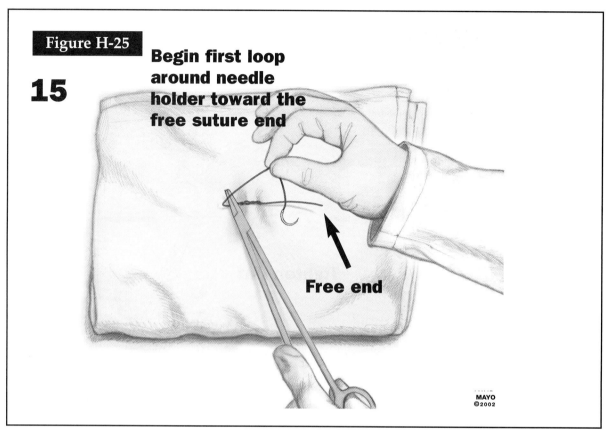

Free end

16

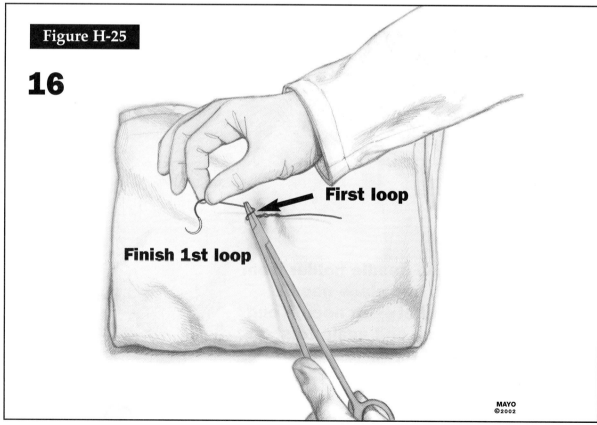

First loop

Finish 1st loop

H. Sutures, Needles and Knots

Figure H-25

17

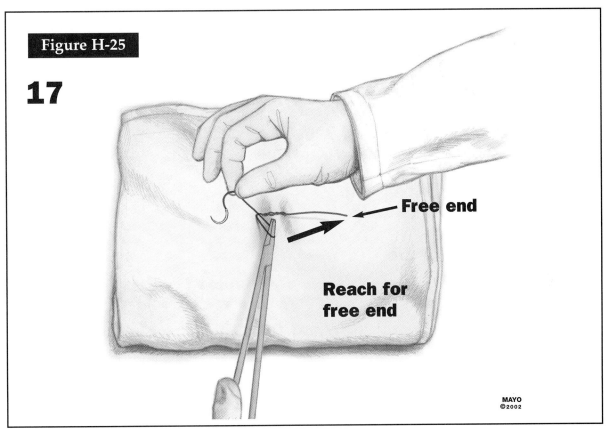

Free end

Reach for free end

MAYO
©2002

Figure H-25

18

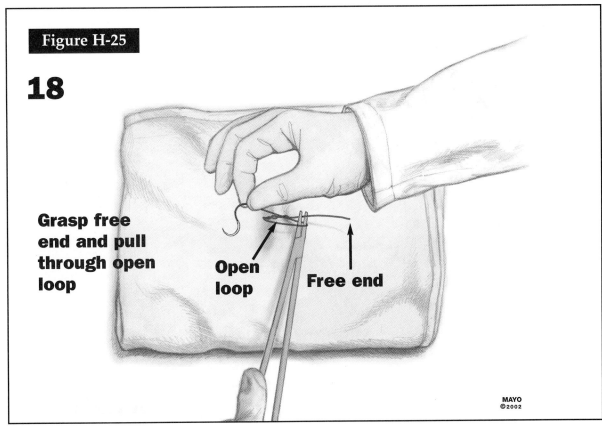

Grasp free end and pull through open loop

Open loop

Free end

MAYO
©2002

H. Sutures, Needles and Knots

Figure H-25

19

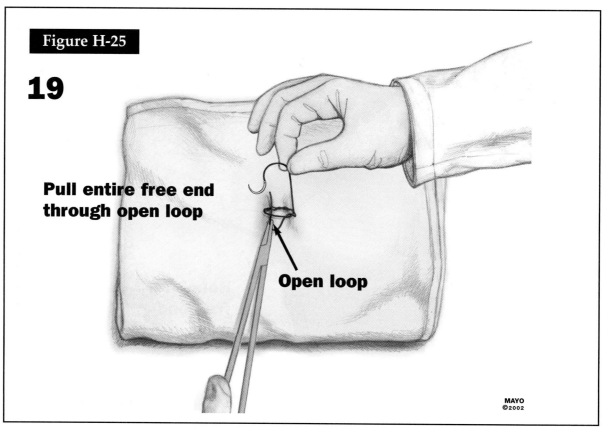

Pull entire free end through open loop

Open loop

MAYO
©2002

Figure H-25

20

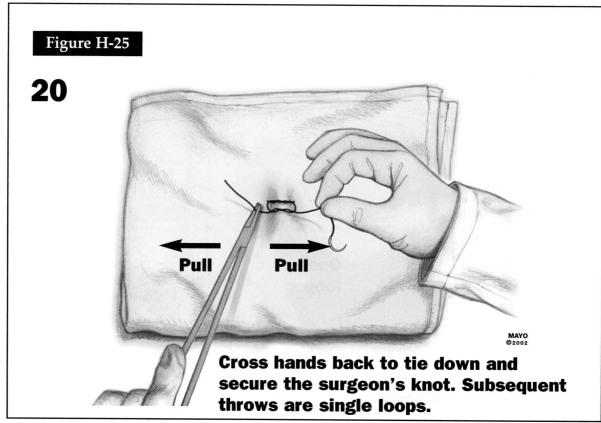

Pull

Pull

MAYO
©2002

Cross hands back to tie down and secure the surgeon's knot. Subsequent throws are single loops.

I. Obtaining Hemostasis

1. The Basics of Hemostasis

The complicated process that stops the bleeding from injured and cut blood vessels is called **hemostasis**. Hemostasis simply refers to the process of stopping bleeding. The human body's response to vascular trauma involves: A) blood vessels and B) blood components.

a. Blood vessels include:
1. Arteries

2. Arterioles

3. Veins

4. Venules

5. Capillaries

When blood vessel injury occurs, the inner lining (the term is endothelial lining) reacts with activation of coagulation. The arteries and arterioles, both which contain smooth muscle layers, also react (vasoconstrict) to reduce blood loss.

b. Blood components include:
1. Plasma 60%

2. Blood cells 40%

  a. Red blood cells (erythrocytes) carry oxygen

  b. White blood cells (leukocytes) digest dead cells, tissue and foreign substances.

  c. Platelets (thrombocytes) help in clotting of the blood.

2. The Coagulation Cascade

The **coagulation cascade** refers to the sequence of chemical reactions that ultimately results in the formation of a fibrin clot **(Figures I-1)**.

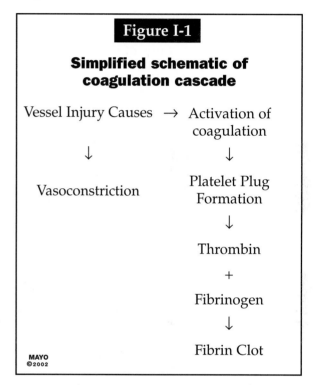

Figure I-1

Simplified schematic of coagulation cascade

Vessel Injury Causes → Activation of coagulation

↓   ↓

Vasoconstriction   Platelet Plug Formation

↓

Thrombin

+

Fibrinogen

↓

Fibrin Clot

MAYO
©2002

The body's normal hemostatic process can be simplified into four discrete sequential phases:

a. Vasoconstriction: Smooth muscle contraction causes vasoconstriction of the arteries and arterioles which reduces blood flow to the injured area.

b. Platelet plug formation: Platelet activation proceeds through various stages that finally results in the formation of a platelet plug.

c. Fibrin clot formation: Because of higher blood pressure in arteries and arterioles, the formation of the platelet plug requires the addition of the coagulation cascade to maintain the strength of a fibrin clot.

d. Fibrinolysis: To control and prevent excessive clotting a process called fibrinoly-

I. Obtaining Hemostasis

sis occurs. In this process the fibrin clot is broken down and allows blood flow through the undamaged blood vessels.

Bleeding is not only the enemy of exposure but it may be extensive enough to produce shock; a life threatening situation for the patient. The diagnosis and treatment of shock is very important but is beyond the scope of this work.

3. Topical Hemostasis

Topical hemostasis acts by chemical and/or mechanical means to stop the bleeding. The body eventually will resorb these topical hemostatic materials from the surgical site.

The general comprehensive class of topical hemostats include:

a. Gelatin
This is usually applied topically. As the gelatin swells it absorbs blood to control oozing. In addition the gelatin adheres to platelets and enhances platelet plug formation.

1. Sponge (Surgifoam®) (**Figures I-2, I-3**).

2. Film (Gelfilm®) (**Figures I-4, I-5**).

b. Cellulose
Oxidized regenerated cellulose (Surgicel ®). The action is similar to gelatin. This material does not fray (**Figures I-6, I-7**).

c. Cotton fiber
Oxidized gauze (Oxycel ®) is similar in action to gelatin. This material has tendency to fray and lint (**Figures I-8, I-9**).

d. Collagen
(Avitene ®) derived from animal (bovine) collagen. Collagen traps platelets and induces the coagulation cascade producing the fibrin clot.

It is supplied as sponge-like sheets, pads, and felt (**Figures I-10, I-11**).

e. Thrombin (topical thrombin USP)
Thrombin derived from animal (bovine) blood. Thrombin accelerates clot formation by quickly (in seconds) converting fibrinogen into a fibrin clot.

It comes as a powder and may be sprinkled on an oozing surface or put into isotonic saline and sprayed on a wound or applied through a **laparoscope**.

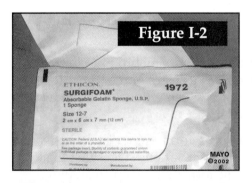
Figure I-2

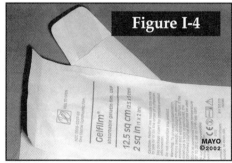
Figure I-4

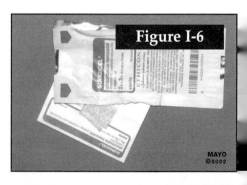
Figure I-6

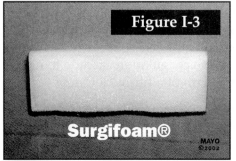
Figure I-3
Surgifoam®

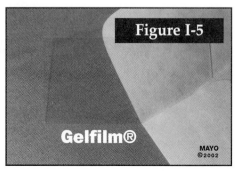
Figure I-5
Gelfilm®

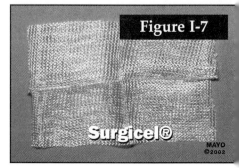
Figure I-7
Surgicel®

I. Obtaining Hemostasis

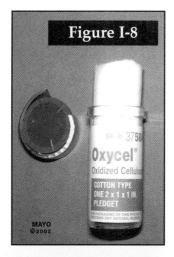

Figure I-8

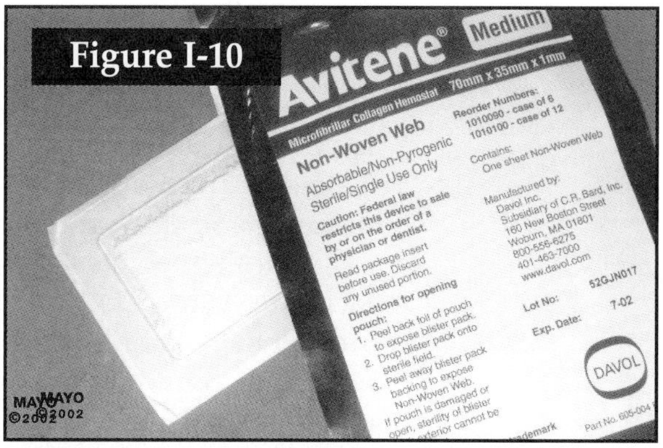

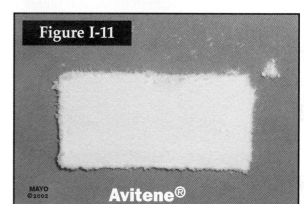

Figure I-10

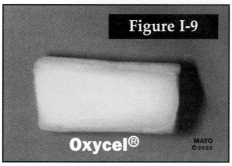

Figure I-9

Oxycel®

Figure I-11

Avitene®

NOTE. NEVER INJECT THROMBIN INTO A VESSEL SINCE DIFFUSE INTRAVAS-CULAR CLOTTING AND DEATH MAY OCCURE! TOPICAL APPLICATION OF THROMBIN ONLY.

f. Fibrin (glues and sealants)
Mixtures of thrombin and fibrinogen bypasses the coagulation cascade and clot formation occurs almost instantaneously.

4. Indications for Use of Topical Hemostatic Agents

Indications for use of topical hemostatic agents are the following:

a. Capillary oozing.

b. Hard to reach areas.

c. Oozing from suture lines .

d. Cerebral spinal fluid (CSF) leaks (especially fibrin glue or sealants).

There are a number of methods used to obtain hemostasis. These are all methods to stop bleeding. **THE SIMPLEST AND MOST DIRECT METHOD TO CONTROL BLEEDING IS BY DIRECT FINGER PRES-SURE ON THE BLEEDING SITE.** The other common methods are free vessel ligature, figure-of-eight stick tie, electrocautery, and bone wax.

I. Obtaining Hemostasis

5. Free Vessel Ligature

Free vessel ligature is tying off vessels that have been clamped in a hemostat. The clamp is held by the assistant, and the surgeon passes the ligature around the hemostat. The assistant then points the tip of the hemostat facing upward. The surgeon loops the suture around the end of the hemostat so that it is encircled around the vessel. A two-hand tie of either a square knot or a surgeon's knot is then performed **(Figures I-12)**. After pulling

down and securing the second throw of the knot, the assistant, at the surgeon's direction, releases the hemostat from the vessel. The surgeon then completes the third throw and secures the knot **(Figures I-13)**.

At least 4 knots should be placed in a vessel ligature unless the surgeon instructs otherwise.

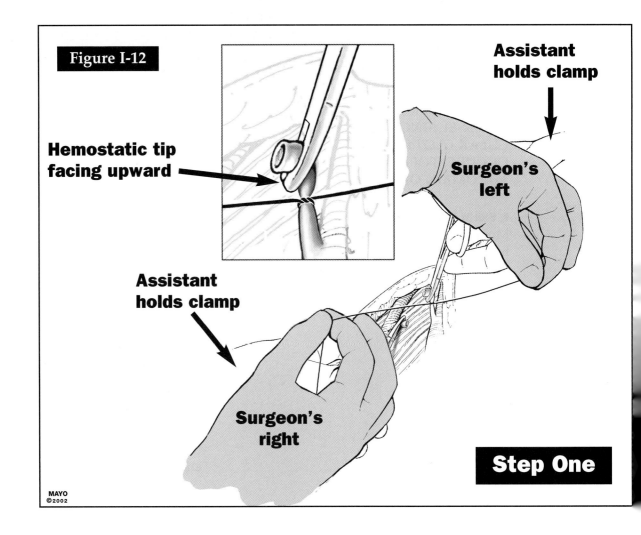

Figure I-12

Hemostatic tip facing upward

Assistant holds clamp

Surgeon's left

Assistant holds clamp

Surgeon's right

MAYO ©2002

Step One

I. Obtaining Hemostasis

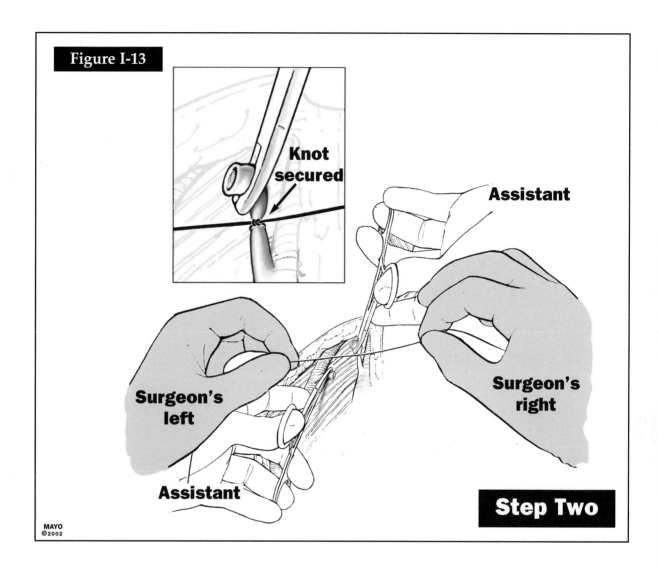

Figure I-13

Knot secured

Assistant

Surgeon's right

Surgeon's left

Assistant

Step Two

MAYO
©2002

I. Obtaining Hemostasis

6. Figure-of-8 Stick Tie

The stick tie is a variation of the free vessel ligature and is useful for larger vessels or tissue pedicles. The stick tie is more secure and less likely to loosen and fall off during the postoperative period. The tissue to be tied is usually held in a hemostat or larger clamp. The needle is passed back and forth through the tissue under the clamp in a figure-of-8 fashion **(Figure I-14, numbers 1-12).**

The first throw is a surgeon's knot **(Figure I-14, number 6)**. The free ends of the suture are then passed around the two sides of the clamp and the knot is completed with subsequent throws **(Figure I-14, numbers 7-12)**.

FIGURE-OF-8 STICK TIE

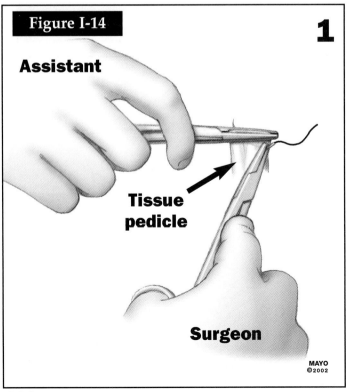

Figure I-14 **1**

Assistant

Tissue pedicle

Surgeon

MAYO
©2002

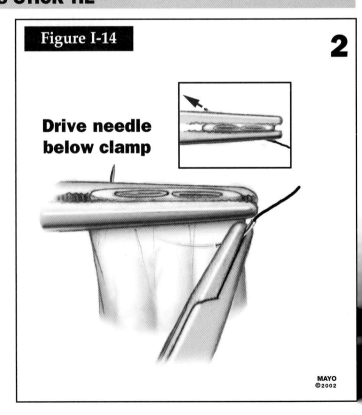

Figure I-14 **2**

Drive needle below clamp

MAYO
©2002

FIGURE-OF-8 STICK TIE

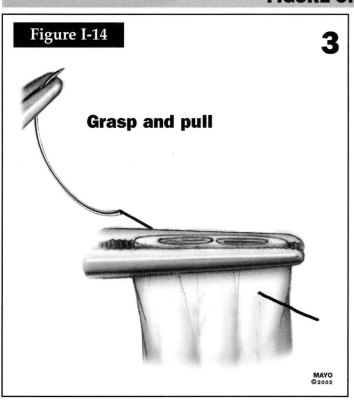

Figure I-14

3

Grasp and pull

MAYO
©2002

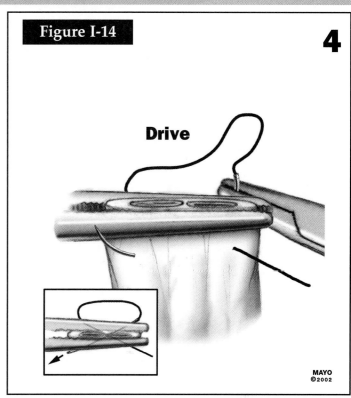

Figure I-14

4

Drive

MAYO
©2002

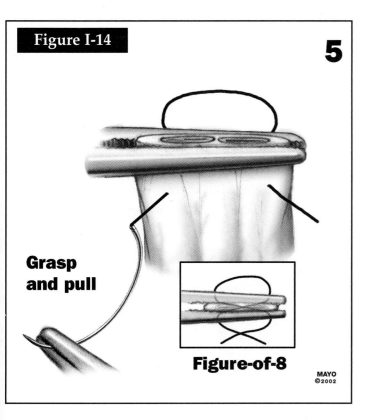

Figure I-14

5

Grasp and pull

Figure-of-8

MAYO
©2002

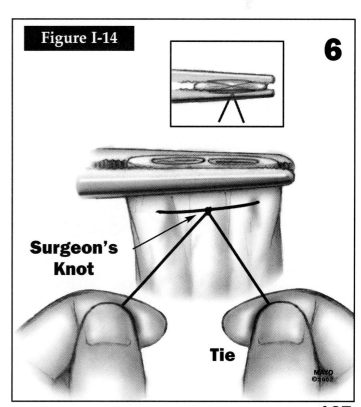

Figure I-14

6

Surgeon's Knot

Tie

MAYO
©2002

I. Obtaining Hemostasis

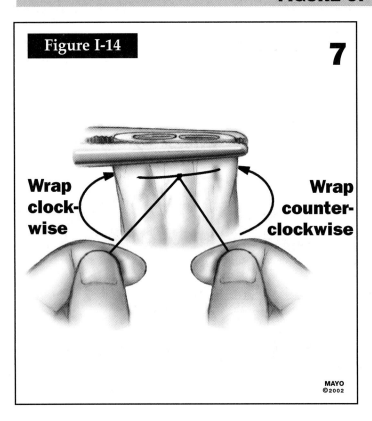

Figure I-14   **7**

Wrap clock-wise

Wrap counter-clockwise

MAYO ©2002

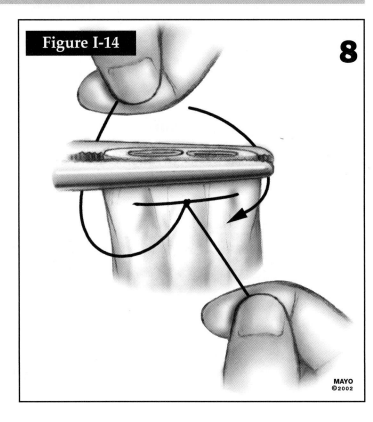

Figure I-14   **8**

MAYO ©2002

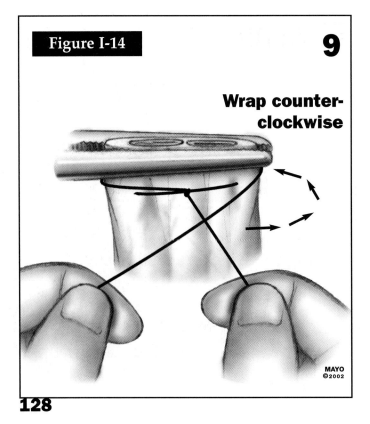

Figure I-14   **9**

Wrap counter-clockwise

MAYO ©2002

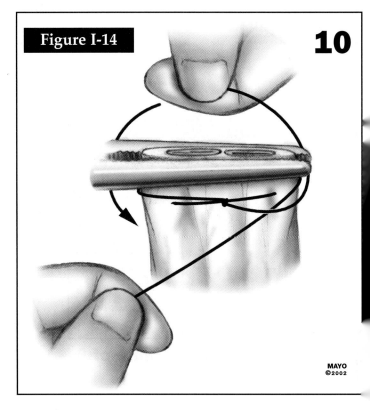

Figure I-14   **10**

MAYO ©2002

I. Obtaining Hemostasis

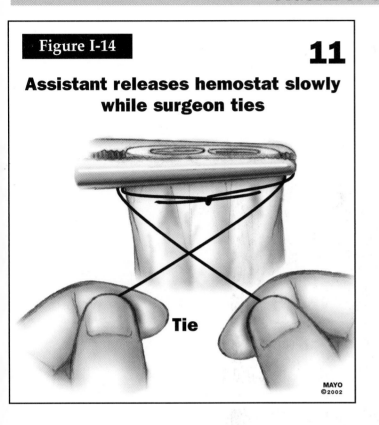

Figure I-14 11

Assistant releases hemostat slowly while surgeon ties

Tie

MAYO
©2002

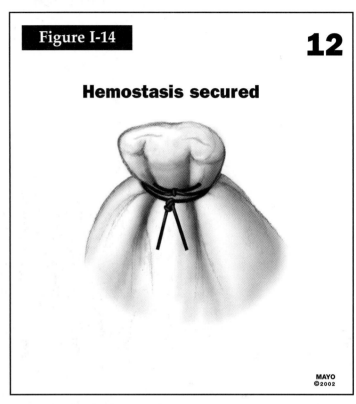

Figure I-14 12

Hemostasis secured

MAYO
©2002

7. Electrocautery

It is faster to cauterize smaller vessels than to tie them off. The surgeon can cauterize the tiny vessels directly. Smaller vessels can also be cauterized by having the assistant hold up the clamped vessel with the hemostat. The surgeon then touches the hemostat with a monopolar cautery. This results in coagulation of the vessel. When the vessel appears adequately coagulated, the surgeon will instruct the assistant to release the hemostat from the vessel. **DO NOT RELEASE THE HEMOSTAT FROM THE VESSEL PRIOR TO DIRECTION FROM THE SURGEON**. If you do release the hemostat from the vessel prior to the coagulation, what will happen? Answer: The vessel will bleed, and the surgeon will be mighty miffed. You will learn not to do that again!

Bipolar cautery, which looks like a forceps, can be used to both grasp and cauterize bleeding vessels directly. This cautery results in burning only the tissue held between the teeth of the instrument. As previously mentioned, there is less transmission of heat and less tissue damage to the surrounding tissues with this technique. The bipolar cautery technique is excellent for stopping bleeding from smaller blood vessels.

I. Obtaining Hemostasis

8. Bone Wax

Bleeding areas of bone can usually be controlled with bone wax. This sterile material is a soft, clay-like substance that is smeared on the bleeding area to occlude the bleeding sites in bone **(Figure I-15-18)**.

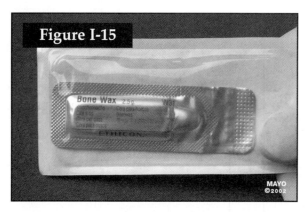
Figure I-15

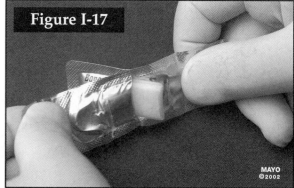
Figure I-17

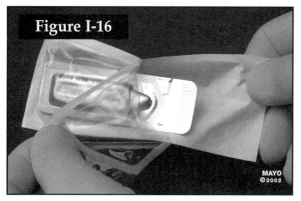
Figure I-16

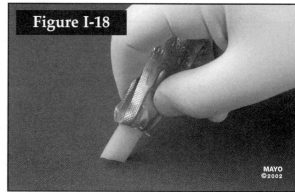
Figure I-18

Quiz

Fill in the blanks below!

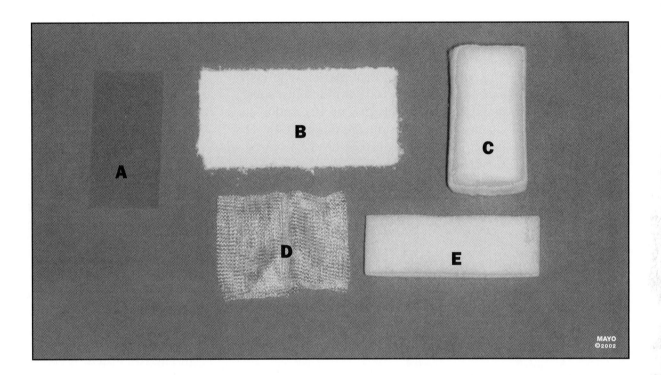

Fill in the blanks and name each product
used for topical Hemostasis.

A. _____

B. _____

C. _____

D. _____

E. _____

Answers

A. Gelatin film, Gelfilm®
B. Collagen, Avitene®
C. Oxidized gauze, Oxycel®
D. Cellulose, Surgicel®
E. Gelatin Sponge, Surgifoam®

J. Wound Closure

1. Principle of Halving

When closing an incision, it is helpful to find the midpoint and place the first suture (central suture) at that site. The suture is placed a few millimeters back from the actual skin edge. The next sutures are then placed in halves on each side of the central suture. Thus, subsequent halving results in complete and even closure of the wound edge **(Figure J-1)**. The principle of halving can be used for both deep closure and skin closure.

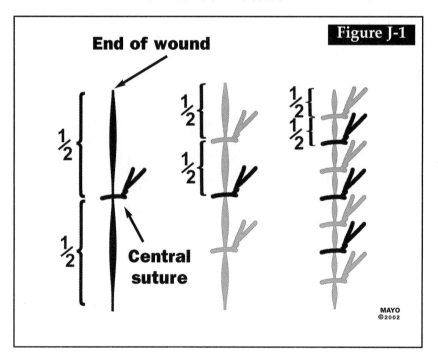

Figure J-1

End of wound

½ ½

Central suture

½ ½ ½

MAYO
©2002

2. Subcutaneous Closure

The anatomic layers of the wound are seen in **Figure J-2**. Note that an intradermal suture placement is also called subcuticular or intracuticular. Large openings in subcutaneous tissue must be closed to prevent dead space in the wound and to take tension off the skin edge. Usually these sutures are placed so that the knots are buried. The first bite is taken away from the surface of the wound edge, deep in the wound, and the needle comes through just below the wound surface **(Figure J-3, 1-4)**. The second bite goes to the opposite side at a corresponding but equal

distance from the surface of the wound edge, and the needle passes deeper into the wound **(Figure J-3:, 5-8)**. The knot is thus buried deep in the wound beneath the wound edge **(Figure J-3, 9,10)**. This prevents extrusion of the knot through the skin.

3. Subcuticular Closure

In some cases the dermal (subcuticular) layer is closed in the same fashion as the subcutaneous layer, using a buried suture technique. The first bite comes away from the wound edge up into the dermis and exits the dermis just below the wound edge. The second bite goes in just below the wound edge on the opposite side and exits at the same distance as in the first bite. The knot is then tied in a buried fashion. This is similar to the subcutaneous closure, except the suture is passed through the dermal (subcuticular) layer. This takes further tension off the skin edge and assists in wound edge eversion, resulting in an improved scar in moderate to high tension wounds. Low tension wounds usually do not necessitate subcuticular closure in this manner.

4. Skin Closure

Once the appropriate subcutaneous and dermal (subcuticular) closures have been done, it is time to close the cut epidermal (skin) layer **(Figure J-3, 11,12)**. A variety of techniques are available to close the incised skin edges. Each technique of skin closure is designed to accomplish the same things: to decrease tension at the epidermal edge during healing, to precisely oppose the skin edges (appoximate and evert) so as to produce the least amount of trauma to the surrounding soft tissues, and to prevent wound infection by direct contamination. All of this promotes healing and will result in a less conspicuous and non-depressed scar.

J. Wound Closure

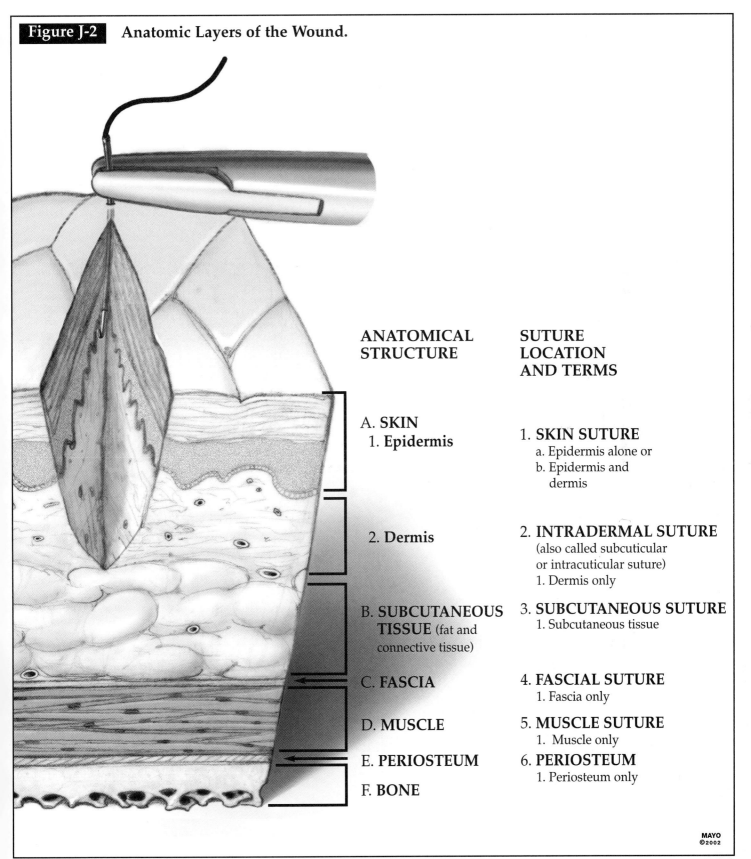

Figure J-2   Anatomic Layers of the Wound.

ANATOMICAL STRUCTURE	SUTURE LOCATION AND TERMS

A. **SKIN**
 1. **Epidermis**
	1. **SKIN SUTURE**
	  a. Epidermis alone or
	  b. Epidermis and
	   dermis

2. **Dermis**	2. **INTRADERMAL SUTURE** (also called subcuticular or intracuticular suture) 1. Dermis only
B. **SUBCUTANEOUS TISSUE** (fat and connective tissue)	3. **SUBCUTANEOUS SUTURE** 1. Subcutaneous tissue
C. **FASCIA**	4. **FASCIAL SUTURE** 1. Fascia only
D. **MUSCLE**	5. **MUSCLE SUTURE** 1. Muscle only
E. **PERIOSTEUM**	6. **PERIOSTEUM** 1. Periosteum only
F. **BONE**	

J. Wound Closure

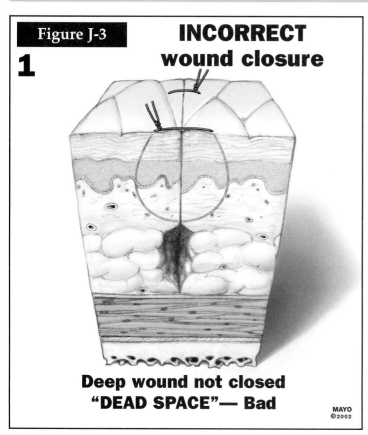

Figure J-3

1

INCORRECT
wound closure

**Deep wound not closed
"DEAD SPACE"— Bad**

MAYO
©2002

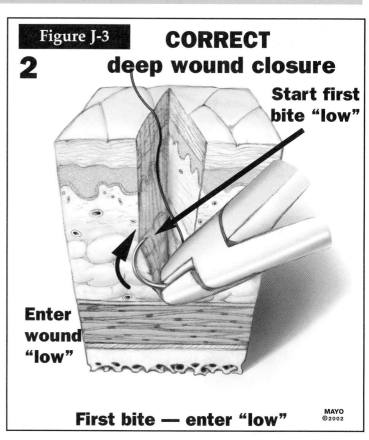

Figure J-3

2

CORRECT
deep wound closure

**Start first
bite "low"**

**Enter
wound
"low"**

First bite — enter "low"

MAYO
©2002

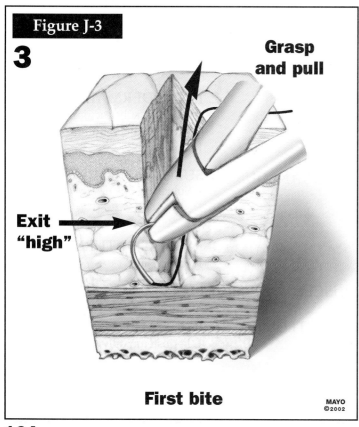

Figure J-3

3

**Grasp
and pull**

**Exit
"high"**

First bite

MAYO
©2002

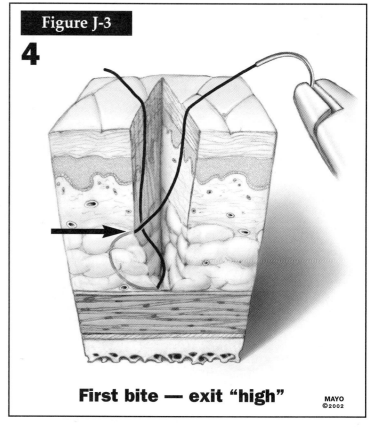

Figure J-3

4

First bite — exit "high"

MAYO
©2002

J. Wound Closure

Figure J-3

5 **Drive**

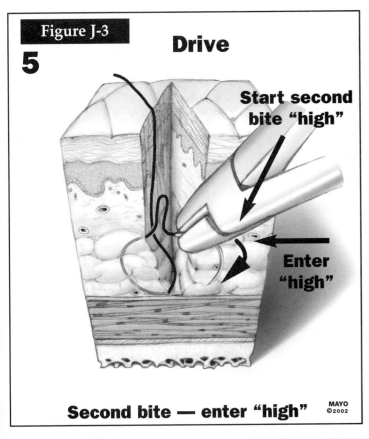

Start second bite "high"

Enter "high"

Second bite — enter "high"

MAYO ©2002

Figure J-3

6 **Grasp and pull**

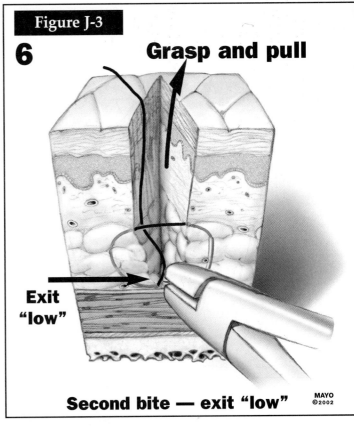

Exit "low"

Second bite — exit "low"

MAYO ©2002

Figure J-3

7 **Tie**

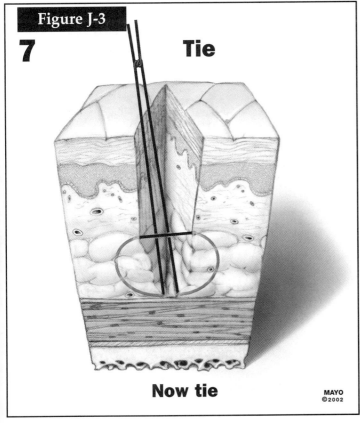

Now tie

MAYO ©2002

Figure J-3

8

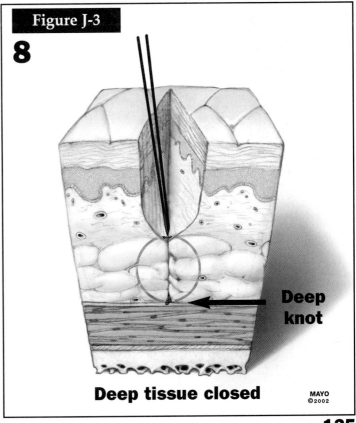

Deep knot

Deep tissue closed

MAYO ©2002

J. Wound Closure

Figure J-3

9

Deep suture cut on knot

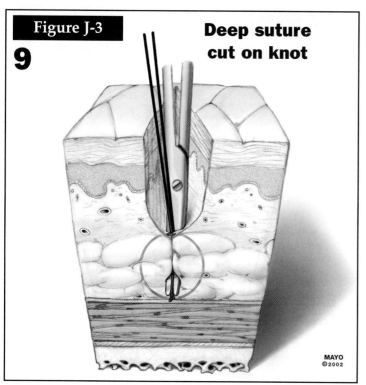

MAYO
©2002

Figure J-3

10

Deep wound closed with suture No dead space

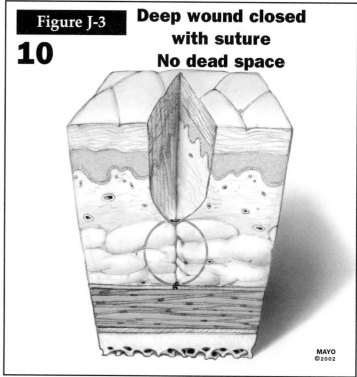

MAYO
©2002

SKIN CLOSURE

Figure J-3

11

Drive

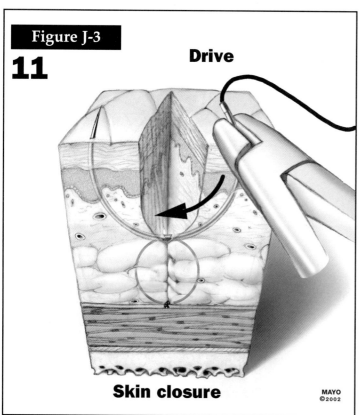

Skin closure

MAYO
©2002

Figure J-3

12

Wound closed correctly

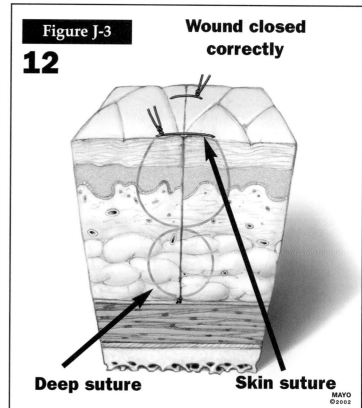

Deep suture

Skin suture

MAYO
©2002

Quiz

Fill in the shaded blanks! See page 133, Figure J-2 for the correct answers.

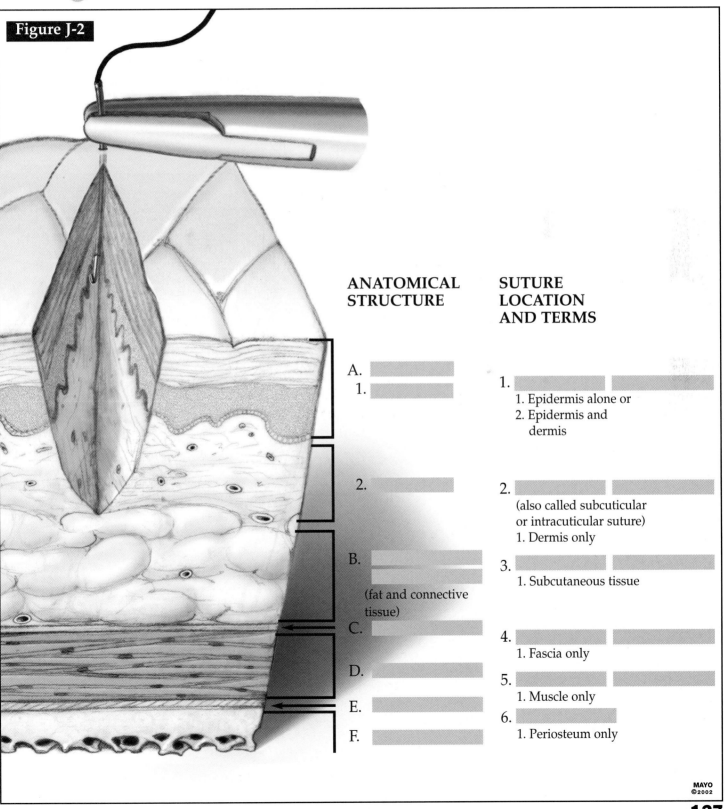

Figure J-2

ANATOMICAL STRUCTURE

A. ▊▊▊▊▊▊
1. ▊▊▊▊▊▊

2. ▊▊▊▊▊▊

B. ▊▊▊▊▊▊
(fat and connective tissue)

C. ▊▊▊▊▊▊

D. ▊▊▊▊▊▊

E. ▊▊▊▊▊▊

F. ▊▊▊▊▊▊

SUTURE LOCATION AND TERMS

1. ▊▊▊▊▊▊ ▊▊▊▊▊▊
1. Epidermis alone or
2. Epidermis and dermis

2. ▊▊▊▊▊▊ ▊▊▊▊▊▊
(also called subcuticular or intracuticular suture)
1. Dermis only

3. ▊▊▊▊▊▊ ▊▊▊▊▊▊
1. Subcutaneous tissue

4. ▊▊▊▊▊▊ ▊▊▊▊▊▊
1. Fascia only

5. ▊▊▊▊▊▊ ▊▊▊▊▊▊
1. Muscle only

6. ▊▊▊▊▊▊
1. Periosteum only

J. Wound Closure

5. Suture Techniques

a. Simple Interrupted Suture

The simple interrupted suture is one of the most commonly used suture techniques. These sutures are useful in essentially any situation. It is a one-bite suture technique. The needle is passed through the skin **PERPENDICULAR** to the skin edge (**Figure J-4**). The needle passes through the entire epidermis and dermis. The second portion of the bite comes out through the opposite side at the same distance from the wound edge and is tied (**Figure J-5,6**). The **goal** is to **approximate** and **evert** the wound edge. The drawings show the technique of the simple interrupted suture (**Figure J-7**). Essentially you want approximated, everted wound edges with suture placement to be as deep as they are wide apart (**Figure J-7**). Note the incorrect and correct (**PERPENDICULAR**) angle of approach to the skin surface. The **PERPENDICULAR** angle of approach helps to evert the wound edges. The sutures are placed equally distant from each other. In addition the depth of the **"bite"** is equal to the distance that the sutures are placed from each other (**Figure J-8**).

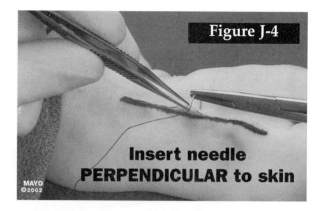

Figure J-4

Insert needle PERPENDICULAR to skin

MAYO
©2002

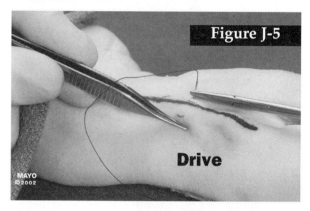

Figure J-5

Drive

MAYO
©2002

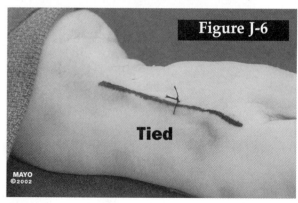

Figure J-6

Tied

MAYO
©2002

J. Wound Closure

Figure J-7

1

INCORRECT

Obtuse angle of approach

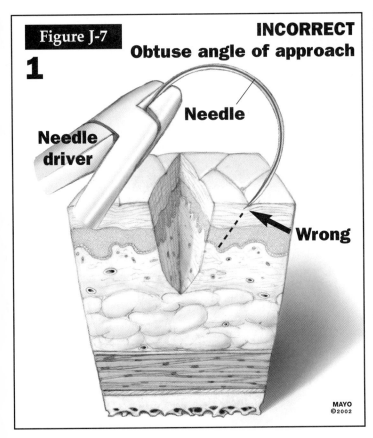

Needle

Needle driver

Wrong

MAYO
©2002

Figure J-7

2

CORRECT

Right angle of approach (90° angle)

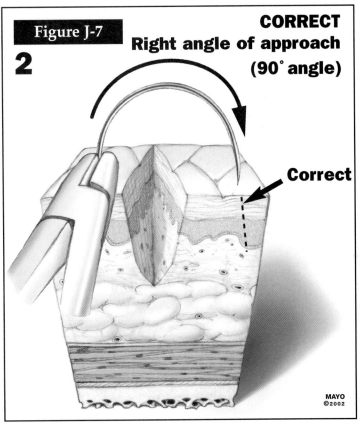

Correct

MAYO
©2002

Figure J-7

3

Drive

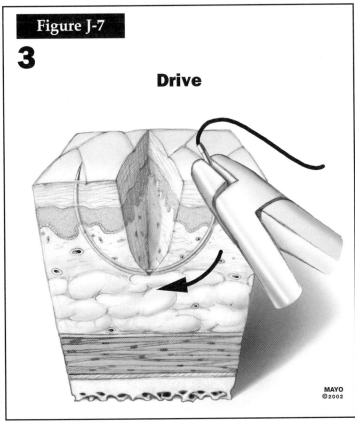

MAYO
©2002

Figure J-7

4

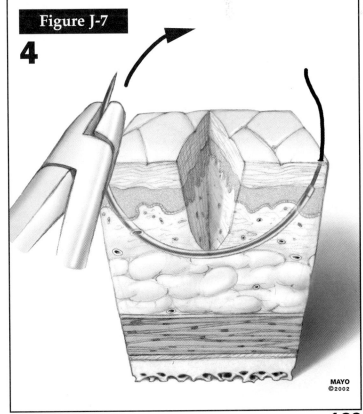

MAYO
©2002

SIMPLE INTERRUPTED SUTURE

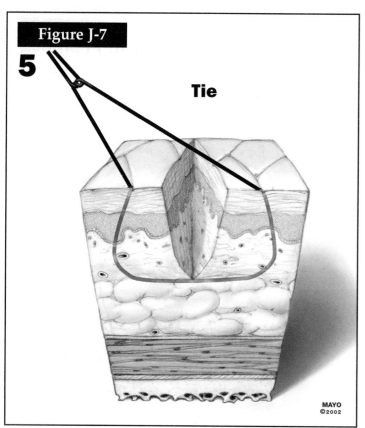

Figure J-7

5

Tie

MAYO
©2002

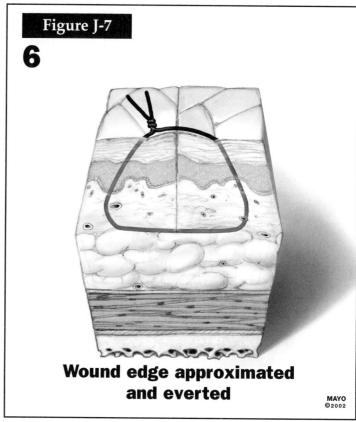

Figure J-7

6

**Wound edge approximated
and everted**

MAYO
©2002

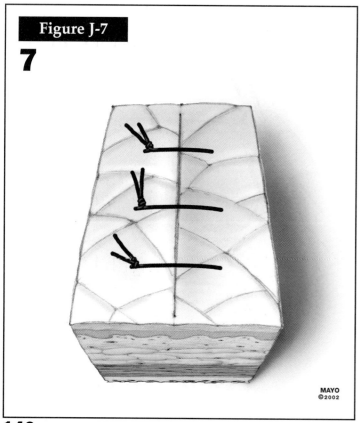

Figure J-7

7

MAYO
©2002

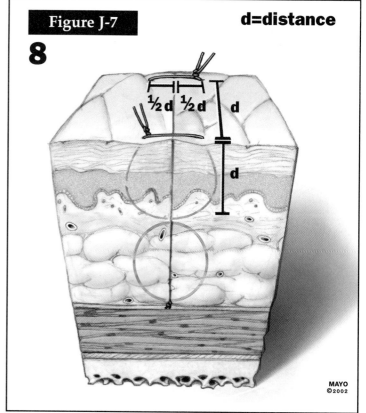

Figure J-7

8

d=distance

½d ½d d

d

MAYO
©2002

Quiz

Fill in the shaded blanks with correct answers! Check out the answers below and see page 139, Figure J-7:1,2 to review the correct answers.

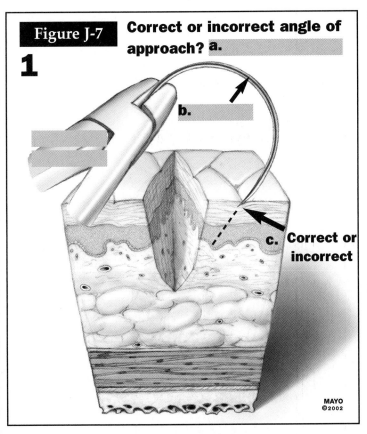

Figure J-7
1

Correct or incorrect angle of approach? **a.**

b.

c. Correct or incorrect

MAYO
©2002

Answers

c. *Incorrect*

b. *Needle*

a. *Incorrect*

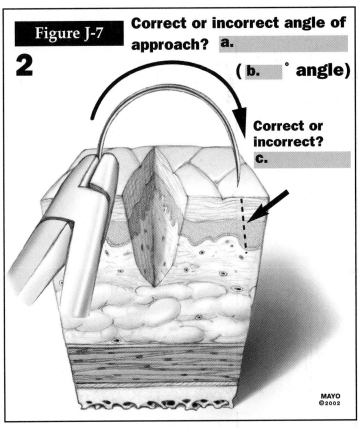

Figure J-7
2

Correct or incorrect angle of approach? **a.**

(**b.** ° angle)

Correct or incorrect?
c.

MAYO
©2002

Answers

c. *Correct*

b. *90°*

a. *Correct*

J. Wound Closure

b. Vertical Mattress Suture

The vertical mattress is a two-bite suture technique. The bites closer to the cut edge of the wound are utilized to precisely approximate and evert the skin edges. The vertical mattress suture is useful when the tissues tend to invert with placement of simple sutures. The vertical mattress gives both excellent eversion and precise skin edge approximation.

The first small bites are placed 1 to 2 mm from the cut edge of wound at the intradermal level **(Figure J-8)**. After the first small bite is precisely placed, the two portions of the suture on each side of the incision are grasped and pulled up **(Figure J-9)**. This provides automatic eversion of the tissue before the next deeper bite. The deeper (second) bite is then placed away from the skin edge starting on the same side of the needle and coming back to the starting side where the free end of the suture is located **(Figure J-10)**.

The suture is then tied on the side of the wound where the wound closure first started **(Figure J-11)**. The deeper second bite helps to reduce tension from the wound edge while the shorter first bite precisely matches the skin edges. The resultant eversion with this suturing technique is excellent and provides less risk of hypertrophic scarring. The drawings show the technical details of the vertical mattress suture **(Figure J-12, 1-6)**.

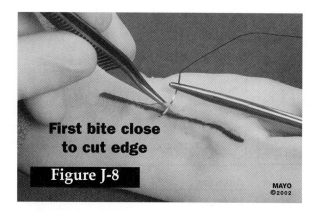

First bite close to cut edge

Figure J-8

MAYO
©2002

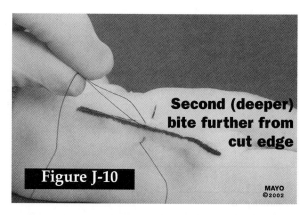

Second (deeper) bite further from cut edge

Figure J-10

MAYO
©2002

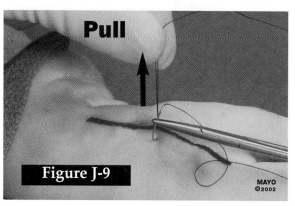

Pull

Figure J-9

MAYO
©2002

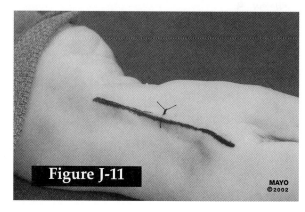

Figure J-11

MAYO
©2002

142

J. Wound Closure

Figure J-12

1

First bite close to cut edge

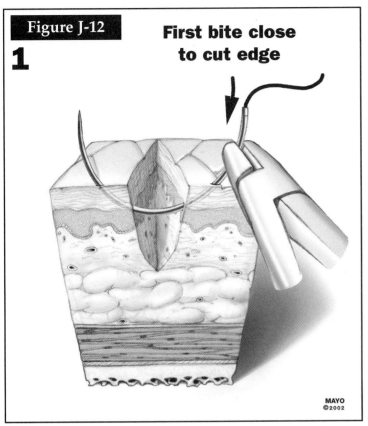

MAYO
©2002

Figure J-12

2

Grasp and pull

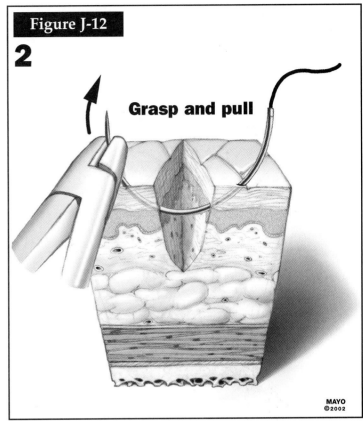

MAYO
©2002

Figure J-12

3

Pull to Evert

Free end

Second bite further from cut edge

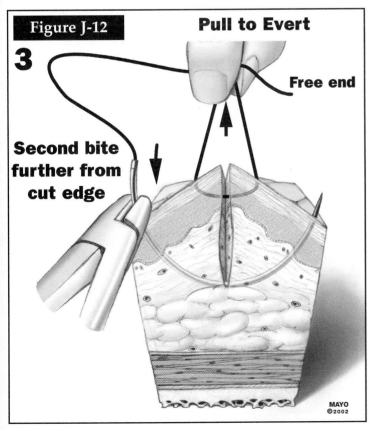

MAYO
©2002

Figure J-12

4

Grasp and pull

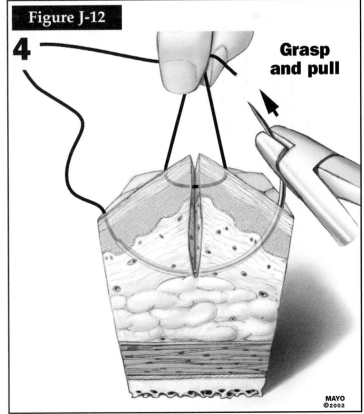

MAYO
©2002

143

J. Wound Closure

Figure J-12

5

Tie

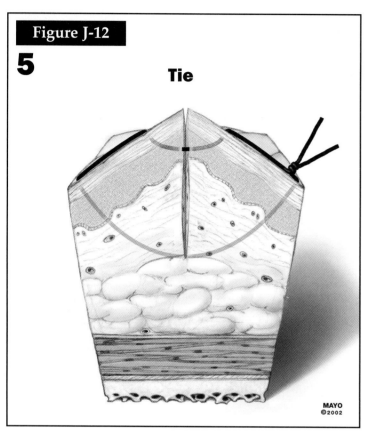

MAYO
©2002

Figure J-12

6

Vertical mattress

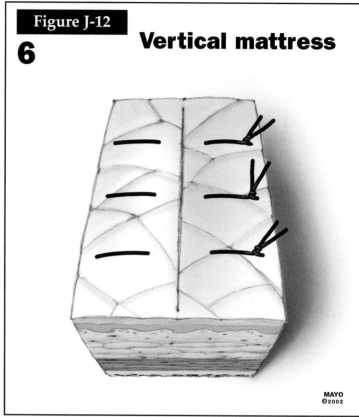

MAYO
©2002

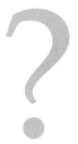

Quiz

The figure to the right is an example of the principle of
_____.

Answer

Halving

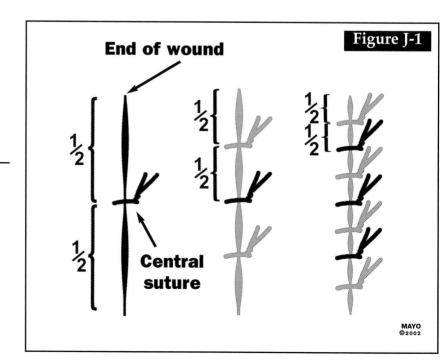

Figure J-1

End of wound

½

½

½

½

½

½

½

Central suture

MAYO
©2002

? Quiz

Fill in the shaded blanks!
See page 35, Figure G-6 for the correct answers.

See page 45, Figure G-29 for the correct answers.

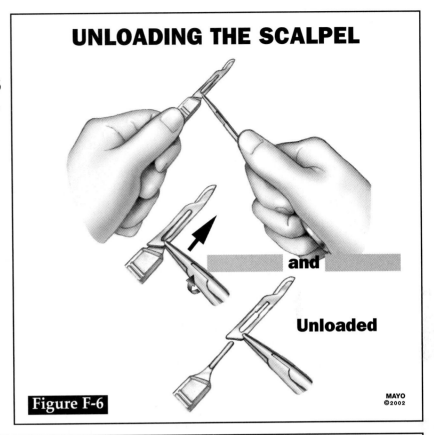

UNLOADING THE SCALPEL

[shaded blank] **and** [shaded blank]

Unloaded

Figure F-6

MAYO
©2002

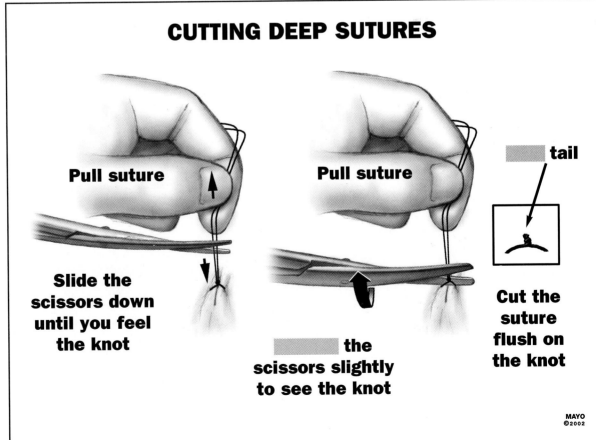

CUTTING DEEP SUTURES

Pull suture

Slide the scissors down until you feel the knot

Pull suture

[shaded blank] **the scissors slightly to see the knot**

[shaded blank] **tail**

Cut the suture flush on the knot

MAYO
©2002

J. Wound Closure

c. Horizontal Mattress Suture

The horizontal mattress suture is also a two-bite suture technique. These two bites are parallel to each other on each side of the wound. The horizontal mattress everts tissue well but does not bring the skin edges precisely together in all cases. Sometimes wide horizontal mattress sutures are placed to take tension off the wound edge. Then a few small simple interrupted sutures or steri-strips are placed at the skin edge to precisely close and approximate the cut wound edges. The horizontal mattress everts as well as the vertical mattress, but is faster to place. The first bite is done exactly as the simple suture **(Figure J-13)**. The second bite is done parallel to the first bite and goes back across the wound edge to end on the same side as the first bite **(Figure J-14)**. The suture is tied on the side of the first bite **(Figure J-15)**. The drawings show the technical details of the horizontal mattress **(Figure J-16, 1-6)**. In both the vertical mattress suture technique and the horizontal mattress suture technique, no suture externally crosses the cut edge of the wound.

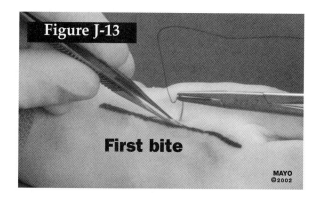

Figure J-13

First bite

MAYO
©2002

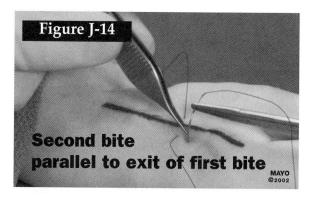

Figure J-14

Second bite
parallel to exit of first bite

MAYO
©2002

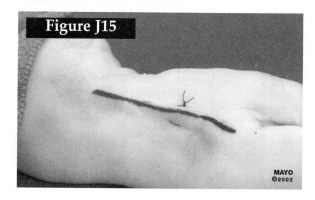

Figure J15

MAYO
©2002

J. Wound Closure

Figure J-16

1 Drive

Free end

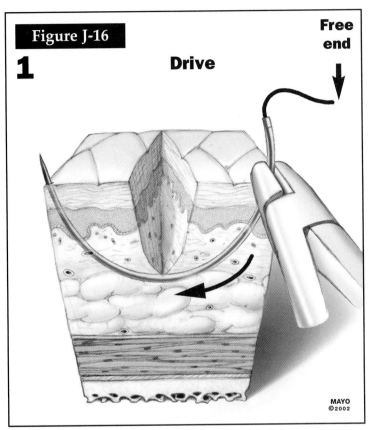

Figure J-16

2 Grasp and pull

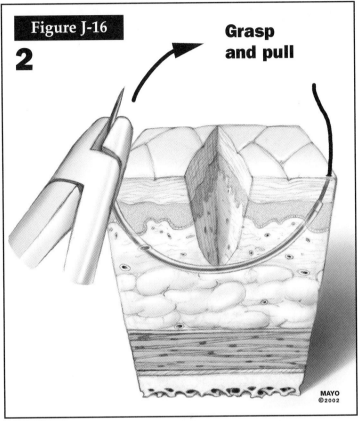

Figure J-16

3 Drive

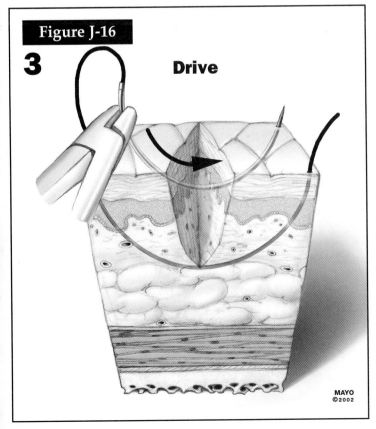

Figure J-16

4 Grasp and pull

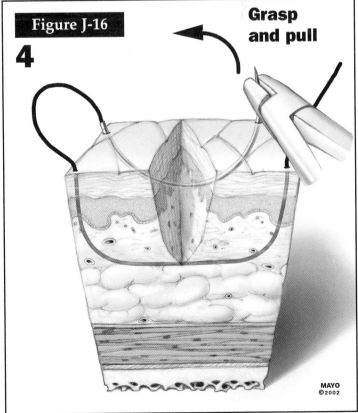

MAYO ©2002

J. Wound Closure

Figure J-16

5 Tie

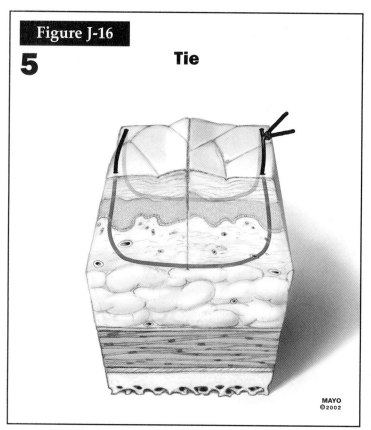

MAYO
©2002

Figure J-16

6 **Horizontal mattress**

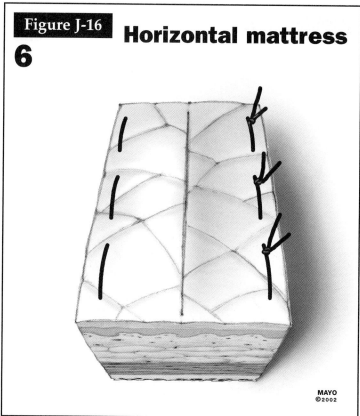

MAYO
©2002

? Quiz

Fill in the blanks! See below for the correct answers.

Name the 3 stages of wound healing

1. Stage 1 - _____ (_____).
2. Stage 2 - _____ .
3. Stage 3 - _____ _____.

Answers

3. *Scar Maturation*
2. *Proliferation*
1. *Inflamation (Vasodilation)*

Quiz

Fill in the shaded blanks! See page 147, Figure J-16 for the correct answers.
Is this is a Horizontal Mattress Suture or Vertical Mattress Suture?

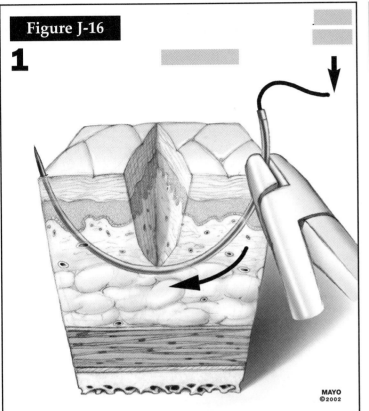

Figure J-16

1

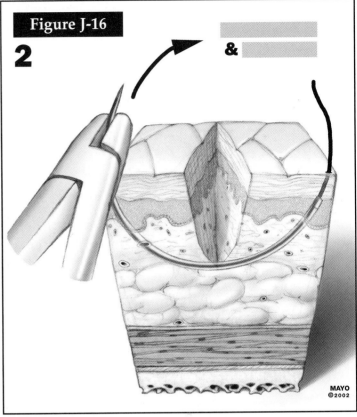

Figure J-16

2

&

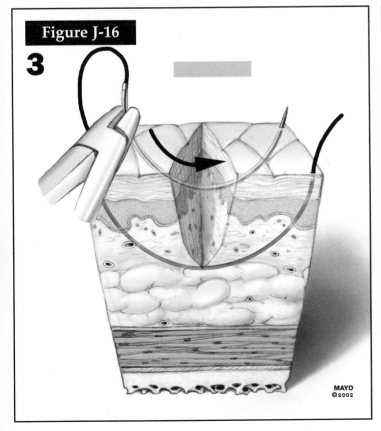

Figure J-16

3

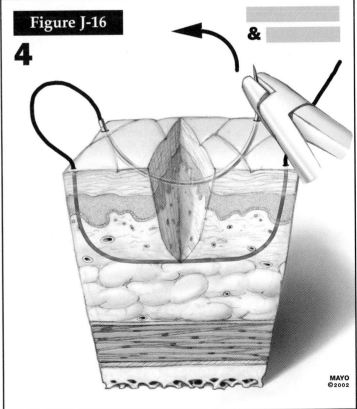

Figure J-16

4

&

J. Wound Closure

d. Running Closure ("Baseball Stitch")

The running closure is often used when the wound's edges easily evert and a long straight incision needs closing. If there is a significant risk of hematoma, the running closure should not be used for the entire length of the incision, as all of the sutures would have to be removed to drain the hematoma.

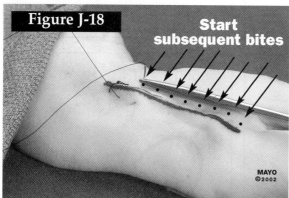

Figure J-17

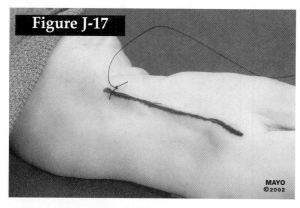

Figure J-18

Start subsequent bites

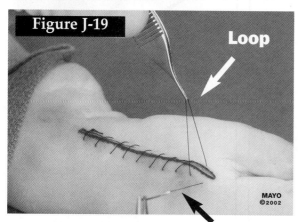

Figure J-19

Loop

Wrap needle end of suture around instrument

If simple interrupted sutures are placed near the ends of the wound, then only these interrupted sutures need be removed for the drainage of a hematoma. The simple running closure or "baseball stitch" is started with a simple suture which is tied off (**Figure J-17**). The free end is trimmed 3 to 4 mm to leave a tail. The end of the suture attached to the needle is not cut. The suturing is now advanced in an equal distance along the cut edge of the wound. The needle "bites" are still perpendicular to the skin edge but the sutures cross the wound externally. Additional simple sutures are placed without tying or cutting the sutures (**Figures J-18, 19**). Constant tension is held on the suture behind the next throw to prevent loosening of the previous sutures. This results in a continuous "baseball stitch" closure. This technique of continuous running closure is a much faster method than the single simple interrupted suturing method.

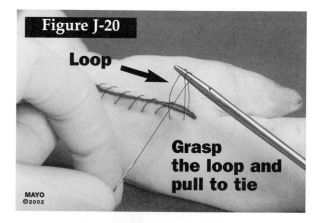

Figure J-20

Loop

Grasp the loop and pull to tie

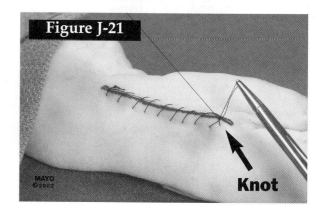

Figure J-21

Knot

150

J. Wound Closure

RUNNING CLOSURE ("BASEBALL STITCH")

At the end, the final throw is placed but not pulled entirely through **(Figure J-19)**. The loop on the next to last throw is utilized as a single strand and the tie done to the loop end of the suture **(Figures J-19, 20, 21)** The free strands are then cut, resulting in 3 tails. Running sutures can be removed by grasping and snipping each subsequent suture and pulling through.

The drawings show the technical details of the running closure **(Figure J-22, 1-11)**.

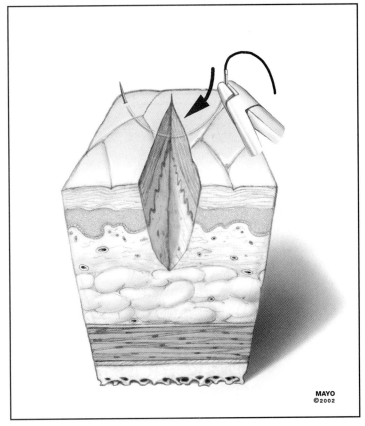

MAYO
©2002

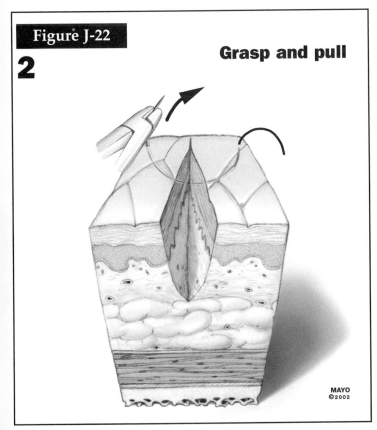

Figure J-22

2

Grasp and pull

MAYO
©2002

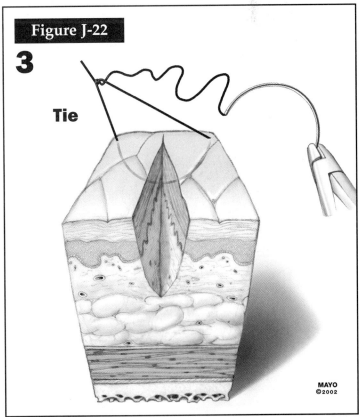

Figure J-22

3

Tie

MAYO
©2002

J. Wound Closure

Figure J-22

4

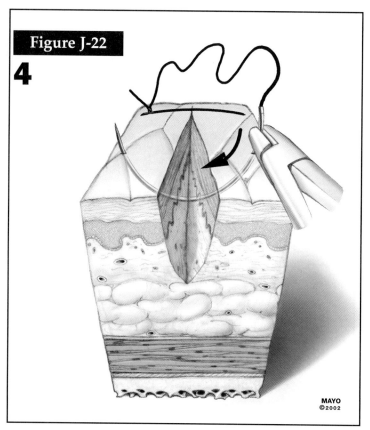

MAYO
©2002

Figure J-22

5

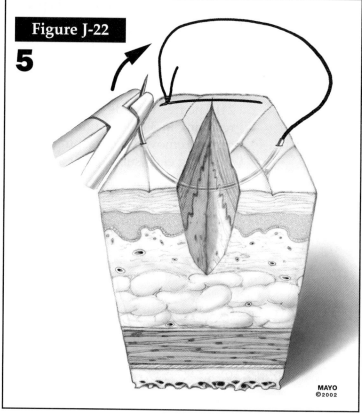

MAYO
©2002

Figure J-22

6

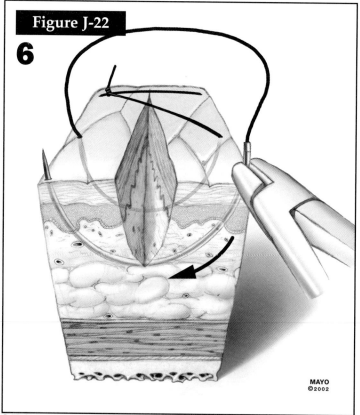

MAYO
©2002

Figure J-22

7

Grasp and pull

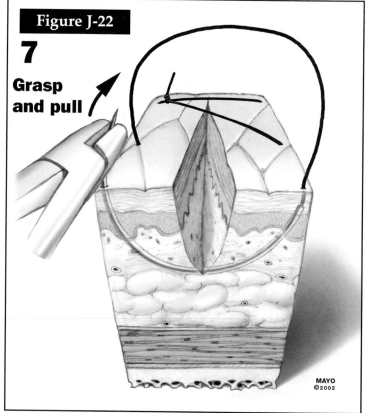

MAYO
©2002

J. Wound Closure

Figure J-22
8

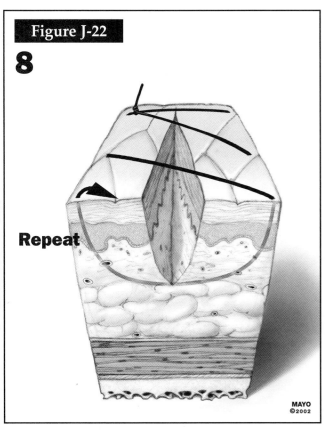

Repeat

MAYO
©2002

Figure J-22
9

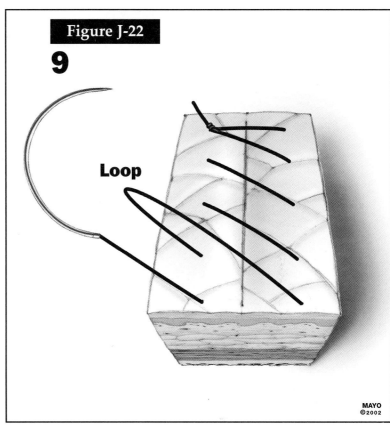

Loop

MAYO
©2002

Figure J-22
10

Tie the loop with the single end

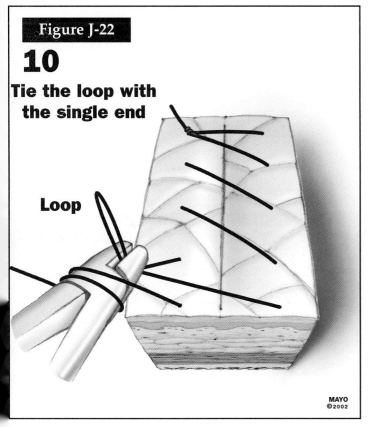

Loop

MAYO
©2002

Figure J-22
11

Start

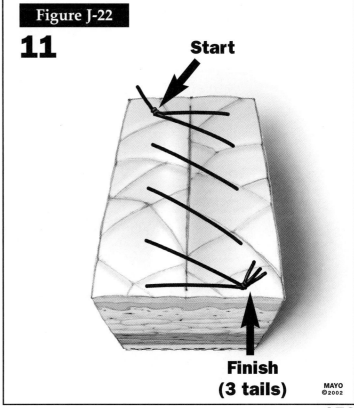

**Finish
(3 tails)**

MAYO
©2002

153

J. Wound Closure

e. Running-Lock Closure

The running-lock closure is a variation of the simple running closure or "baseball stitch." With this technique, the suture is LOCKED prior to placement of the next simple suture **(Figures J-24, 25)**. This results in significantly more tissue eversion. This technique also reduces the skin tension more than the running closure. Thus, in cases where the wound edges tend to invert during closure, or where there is moderate tension, a running-lock closure is a better choice than a simple running closure. In addition, it is easier to remove, as the interdigitations can each be cut away from the cut wound edge. The first and last tie are the same as in the simple running closure **(Figure J-26)**. The drawings show the technical details of the running-lock closure **(Figure J-27, 1-11)**.

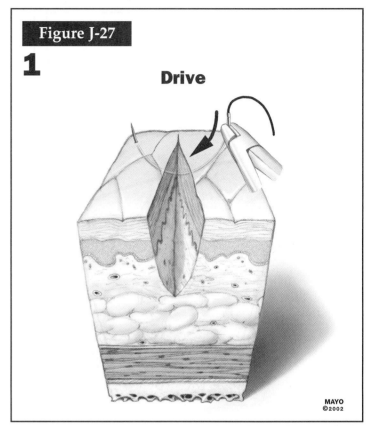

Figure J-27

1

Drive

MAYO
©2002

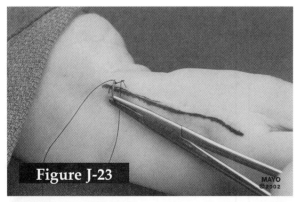

Figure J-23

MAYO
©2002

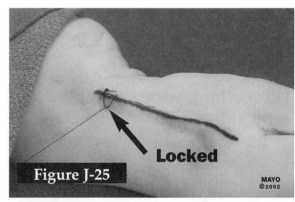

Locked

Figure J-25

MAYO
©2002

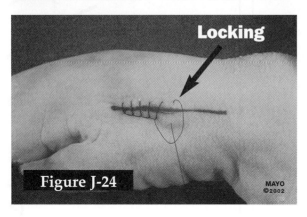

Locking

Figure J-24

MAYO
©2002

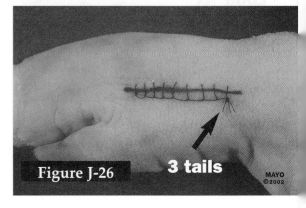

Figure J-26

3 tails

MAYO
©2002

J. Wound Closure

Figure J-27

2

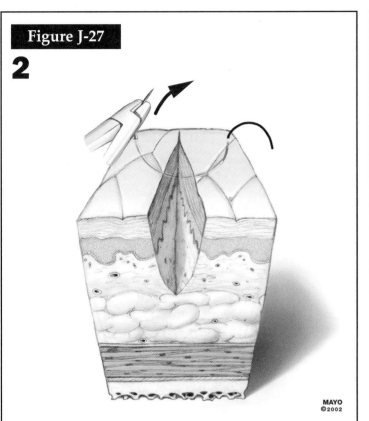

MAYO
©2002

Figure J-27

3

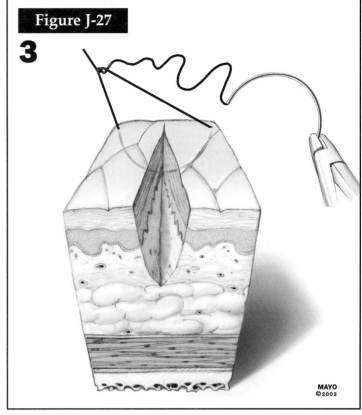

MAYO
©2002

Figure J-27

4

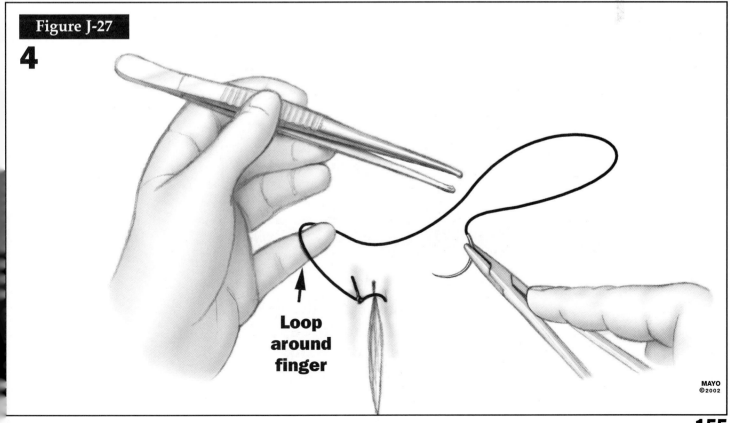

Loop around finger

MAYO
©2002

J. Wound Closure

Figure J-27

5

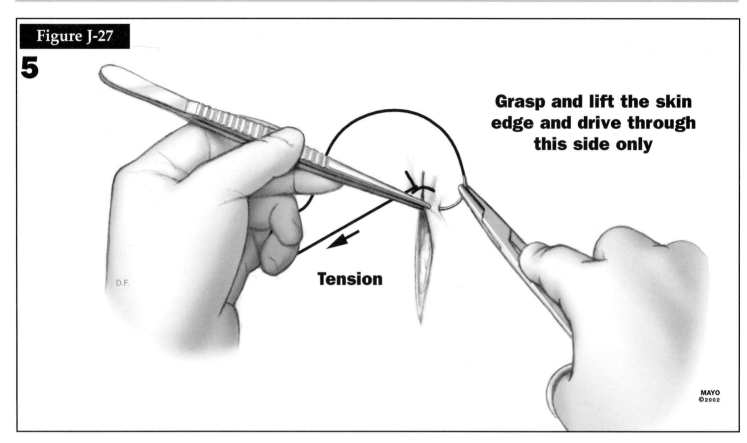

Grasp and lift the skin edge and drive through this side only

Tension

D.F.

MAYO
©2002

Figure J-27

6

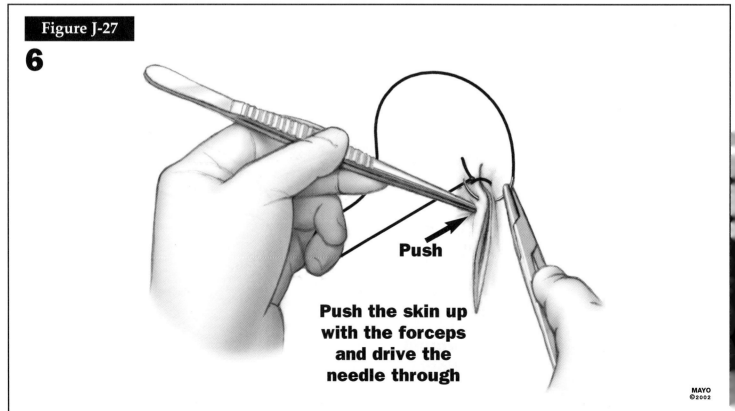

Push

Push the skin up with the forceps and drive the needle through

MAYO
©2002

J. Wound Closure

Figure J-27

7

Bring the loop down over the needle

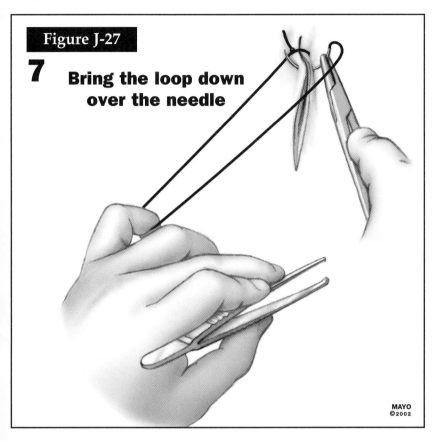

MAYO
©2002

Figure J-27

8

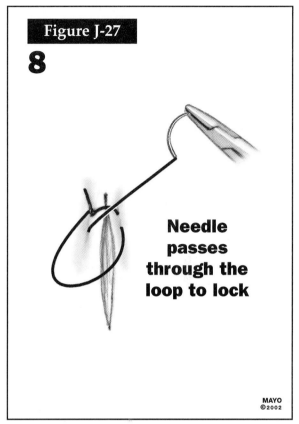

Needle passes through the loop to lock

MAYO
©2002

Figure J-27

9

Repeat steps 4-8

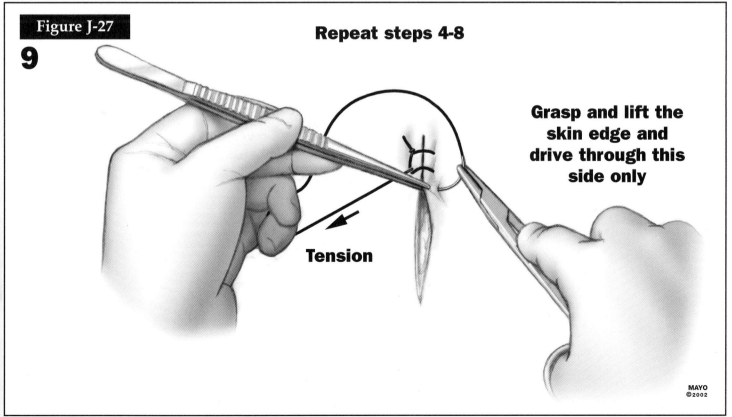

Grasp and lift the skin edge and drive through this side only

Tension

MAYO
©2002

J. Wound Closure

Figure J-27

10

Wrap needle end of suture around needle driver, grasp loop and pull to tie

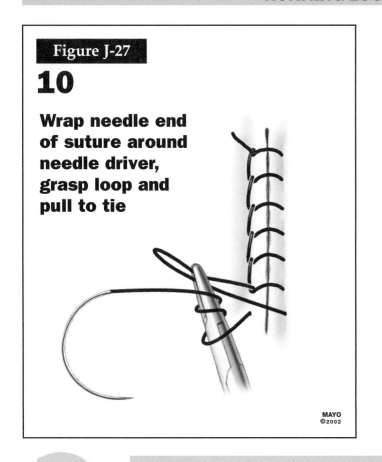

MAYO
©2002

Figure J-27

11

Running lock

Finish
(3 tails)

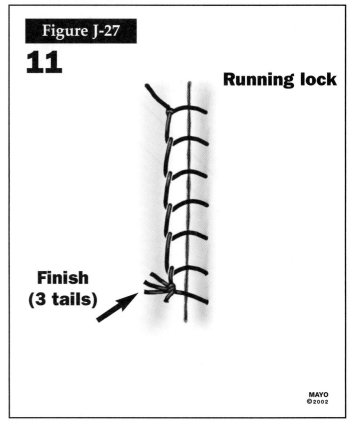

MAYO
©2002

Quiz

Fill in the blanks! See answers below and check out Table H-5, page 61.

Typical suture choices (Suture size and suture material)

Site	Deep Layers	Suture Materials	Skin Layers	Suture Materials
1. Scalp	2-0 to _____	_____	4-0 to _____	_____
2. Face	3-0 to _____	_____	5-0 to _____	_____
3. Trunk	2-0 to _____	_____	2-0 to _____	_____
4. Limbs	2-0 to _____	_____	3-0 to _____	_____

Answers

Site	Deep Layers	Suture Materials	Skin Layers	Suture Materials
1. Scalp	2-0 to 4-0	Absorbable	4-0 to 5-0	Nylon, polypropylene or staples
2. Face	3-0 to 5-0	Absorbable	5-0 to 6-0	Nylon, polypropylene or plain gut.
3. Trunk	2-0 to 3-0	Absorbable	2-0 to 4-0	Nylon, polypropylene or staples
4. Limbs	2-0 to 4-0	Absorbable	3-0 to 5-0	Nylon, polypropylene or staples

Quiz

Fill in the shaded blanks! See page 151. Figure J-22 for the correct answers.
Is this is a Running Closure ("Baseball Stitch") or a Running-lock Closure?

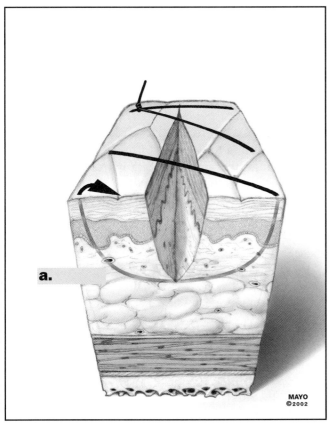

a.

MAYO
©2002

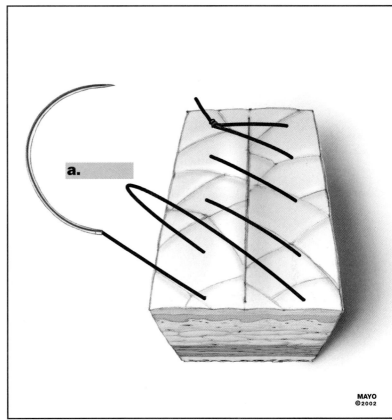

a.

MAYO
©2002

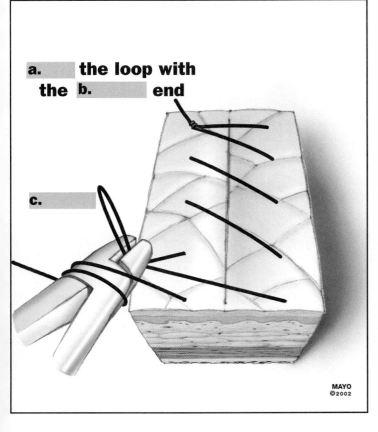

a.   **the loop with**
the b.   **end**

c.

MAYO
©2002

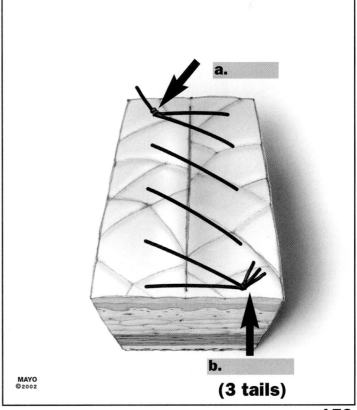

a.

b.

(3 tails)

MAYO
©2002

J. Wound Closure

f. Running Intracuticular (Intradermal) Closure

The running intracuticular closure minimizes penetration of the skin with the needle. This closure is also termed subcuticular or **running intradermal** since it is in the dermis. This is especially useful in keloid patients where needle holes in the skin may stimulate excessive scar formation. It is also useful in children, since removal is quick and easy compared to all other suture techniques. The needle is placed as a first bite single suture technique approximately 1/2 centimeter to 1 centimeter **from the apex** of the wound **(Figure J-28)**. It is then brought into the apex of the wound in the intracuticular (dermal) layer. Multiple intracuticular bites are then placed opposite each other **(Figures J-29, 30)**. There is no penetration of the epidermis (skin) except for the first and last bite. If the incision is long (longer than 3 centimeters), then an intermediate bite is used to place a **surface loop**, which facilitates suture removal.

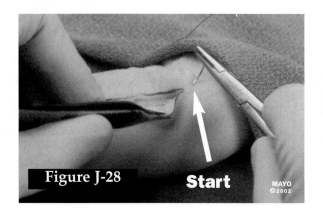

Figure J-28   Start

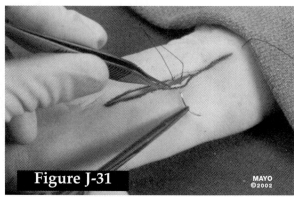

Figure J-31

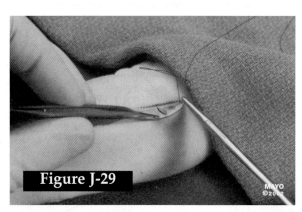

Figure J-29

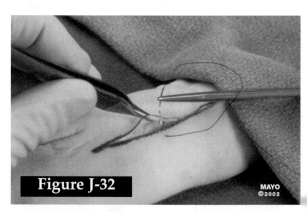

Figure J-32

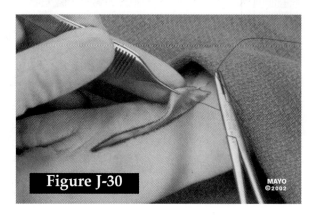

Figure J-30

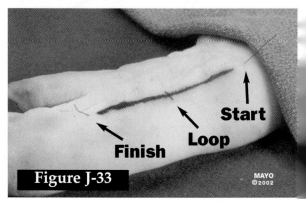

Figure J-33   Start   Loop   Finish

J. Wound Closure

Figures J-31-33 shows the placement of the surface loop midway along the length of incision. The needle is drawn back and forth and a loop is brought out every few centimeters (2-3 centimeters) so that the suture can be easily removed without suture fracture **(Figures J-31-33)**. This loop is brought out through the skin approximately 1/2 centimeter from the skin edge **(Figure J-33)**.

Upon reaching the opposite end of the wound, the needle is placed past the apex of the wound edge and brought out the skin in a similar fashion to the starting side. Typically, with an intracuticular closure, the wound is reinforced with steri-strips or dermabond® which can help reduce tension on the wound. The drawings show the technical details of the running intracuticular closure **(Figure J-34, 1-12)**.

RUNNING INTRACUTICULAR (INTRADERMAL) CLOSURE

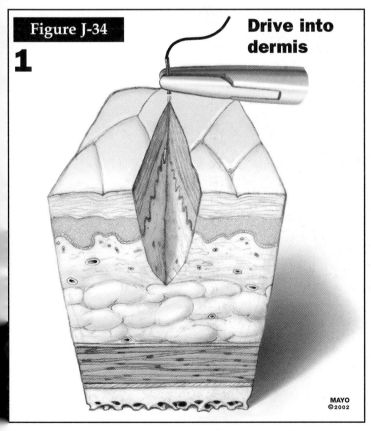

Figure J-34

1

Drive into dermis

MAYO
©2002

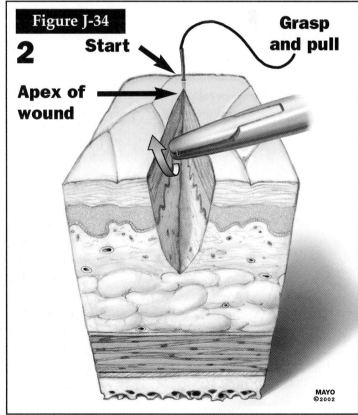

Figure J-34

2

Start

Apex of wound

Grasp and pull

MAYO
©2002

J. Wound Closure

Figure J-34

3

Drive into dermis on left

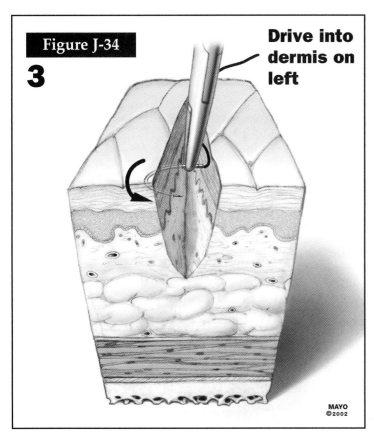

MAYO
©2002

Figure J-34

4

Grasp and pull

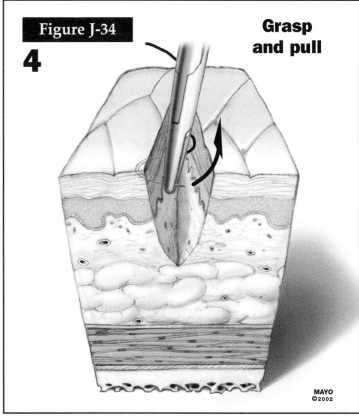

MAYO
©2002

Figure J-34

5

Start

Pull

Apex of wound

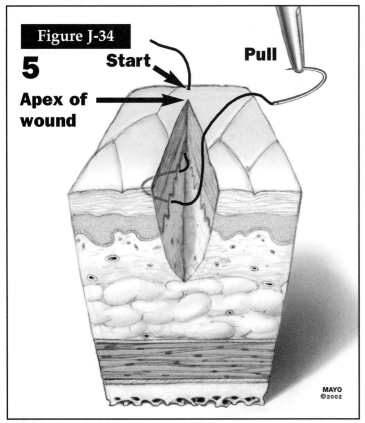

MAYO
©2002

Figure J-34

6

Drive to start loop

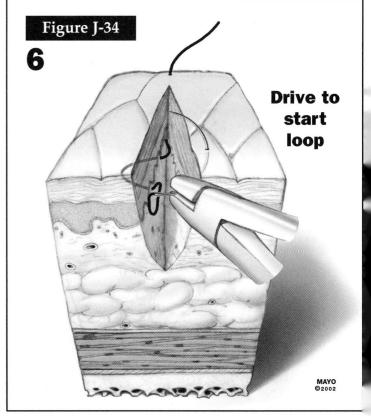

MAYO
©2002

J. Wound Closure

Figure J-34

7

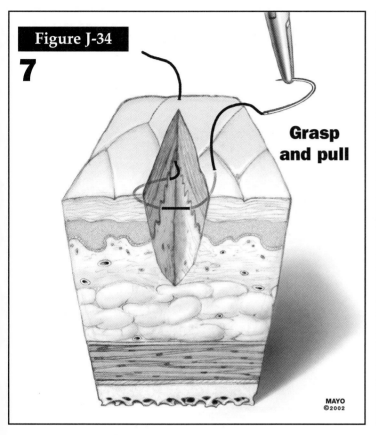

Grasp and pull

Figure J-34

8

Drive to finish loop

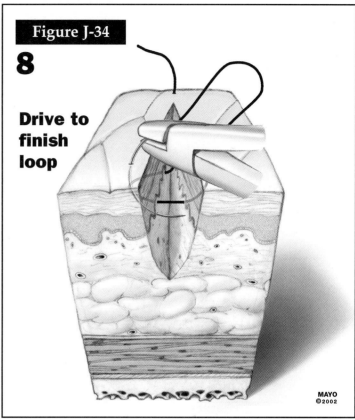

MAYO
©2002

Figure J-34

9

Loop

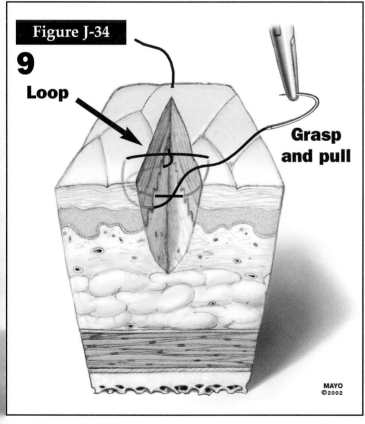

Grasp and pull

MAYO
©2002

Figure J-34

10

Drive into dermis

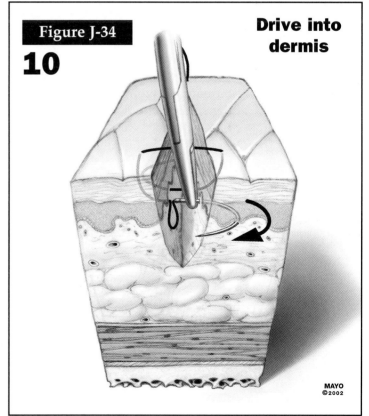

MAYO
©2002

J. Wound Closure

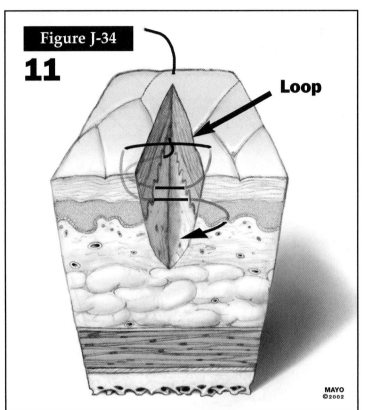

Figure J-34

11

Loop

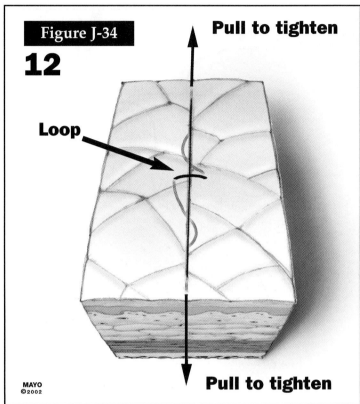

Figure J-34

12

Pull to tighten

Loop

Pull to tighten

MAYO ©2002

Since the ends of the running intracuticular (intradermal) suture are not tied, they are secured by taping the suture ends to prevent loosening. To remove the running intracuticular (intradermal) suture cut at the loop and then pull each end of the suture and it should slide out easily.

g. Purse String Suture

The purse string suture is useful for closing together the edges of a wound where central tissue loss has occurred. Though the edge is irregular at closure the technique may minimize the need for a later local flap or another (revision) surgery. Purse string sutures are especially useful in patients with tissue loss who are not concerned with an optimal cosmetic result. The purse string suture is demonstrated in **Figures J-35, 1-8**.

J. Wound Closure

Figure J-35

1

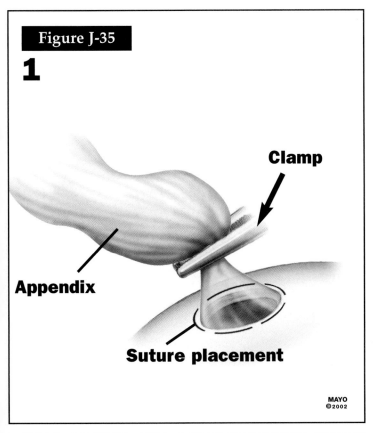

Clamp

Appendix

Suture placement

MAYO
©2002

Figure J-35

2

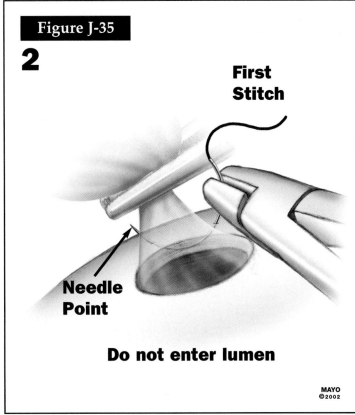

First Stitch

Needle Point

Do not enter lumen

MAYO
©2002

Figure J-35

3

Grasp and pull

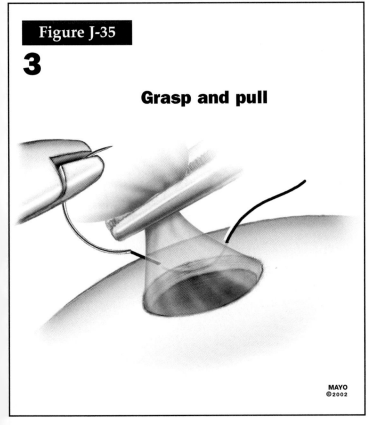

MAYO
©2002

Figure J-35

4

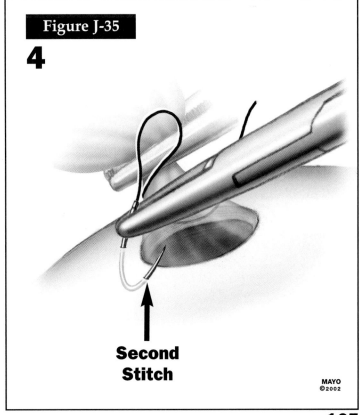

Second Stitch

MAYO
©2002

PURSE STRING SUTURE

Figure J-35

5

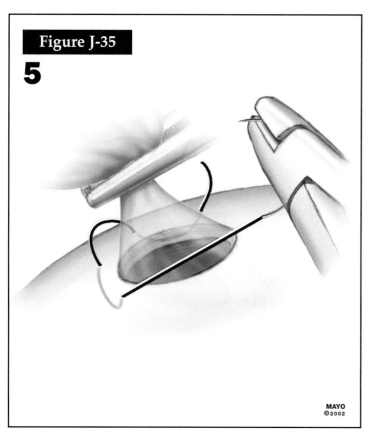

Figure J-35

6

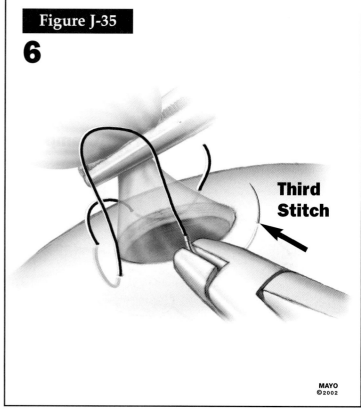

Third Stitch

Figure J-35

7

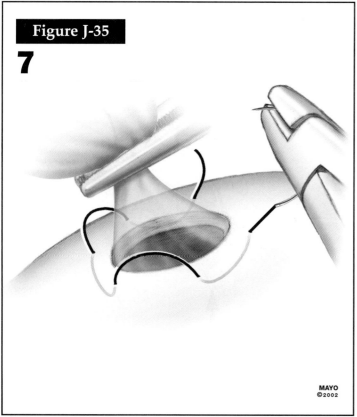

Figure J-35

8

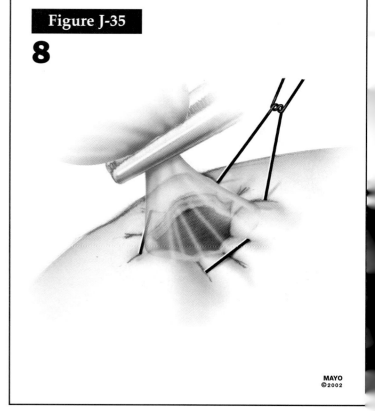

PURSE STRING SUTURE

Figure J-35
9

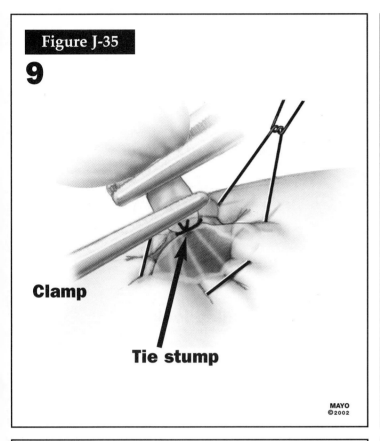

Clamp

Tie stump

MAYO
©2002

Figure J-35
10

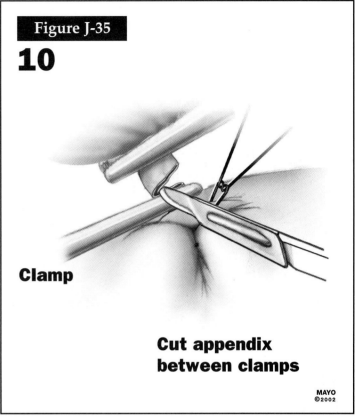

Clamp

Cut appendix between clamps

MAYO
©2002

Figure J-35
11

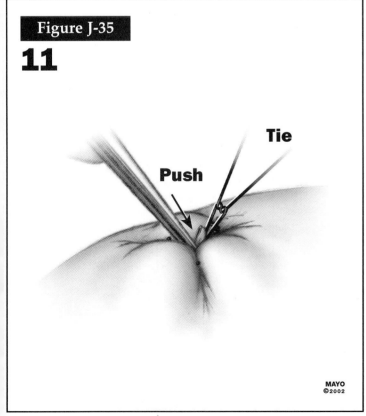

Tie

Push

MAYO
©2002

Figure J-35
12

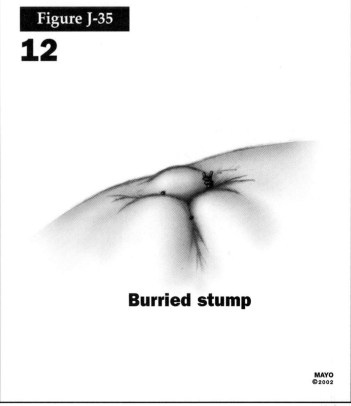

Burried stump

MAYO
©2002

J. Wound Closure

A. Simple interrupted

B. Vertical mattress

C. Horizontal mattress

D. Running (baseball stitch)

E. Running lock

F. Running intracuticular (intradermal)

G. Running intracuticular (intradermal) with surface loop

H. Purse string

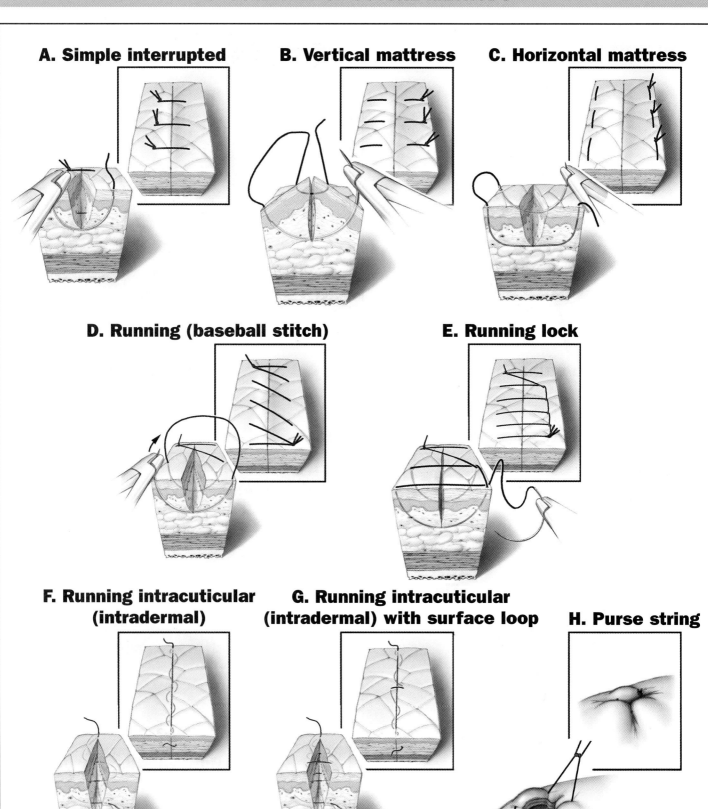

MAYO
©2002

J. Wound Closure

7. Non-Suturing Techniques

The non-suturing techniques to close wounds include a) staples, b) skin adhesives and c) tapes.

a. Staples

The staple closure is used for large wounds that are not on the face. Stapling is especially useful for closure of incisions in hair-bearing skin (scalp). The disposable staple gun is held like a normal hand-held stapler **(Figure J-36)**. The wound edge still needs to be everted manually. Each edge is typically picked up with a forceps, everted and precisely lined up **(Figure J-37)**. The surgeon then places the staples to close the wound while the first assistant advances the forceps, everting the edges of the wound. This technique is continued until the entire wound is everted and closed with staples **(Figure J-38)**.

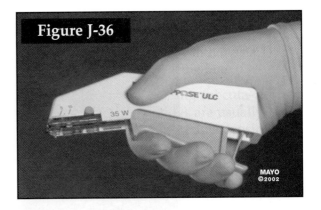

Figure J-36

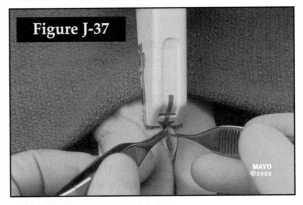

Figure J-37

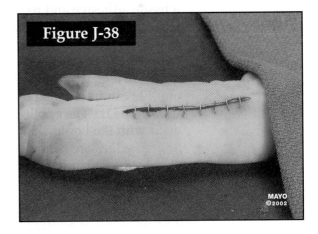

Figure J-38

c. Steri-Strips

Steri-strips are used to close very low tension wounds. They help keep the wound edges together **(Figures J-45 - J-49)**. Steri-strips can also be useful to help keep the wound covered and its edges together even after skin sutures have been placed. They can be especially helpful after intracuticular closures.

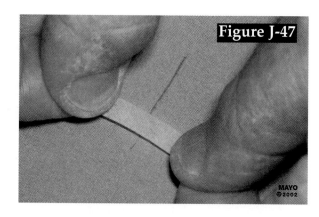

Figure J-47

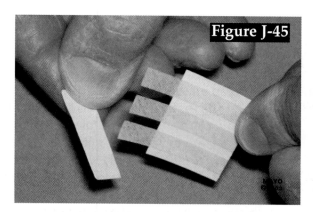

Figure J-45

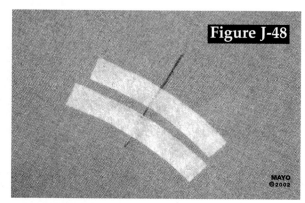

Figure J-48

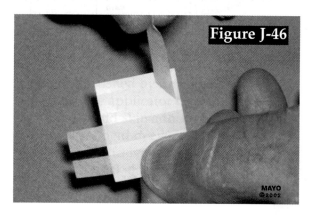

Figure J-46

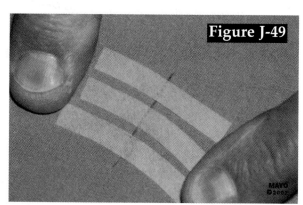

Figure J-49

J. Wound Closure

8. Drains

Drains are used to help close the dead space in a wound by removing serum and blood from the deep portions of the wound. Nonsuction drains **(Figure J-50)** depend on gravity, while suction drains are attached to a bulb or suction unit **(Figure J-51, 52)**. The drains can be cut to various lengths and fixed to the skin with suture or tape. **(Figure J-53)**.

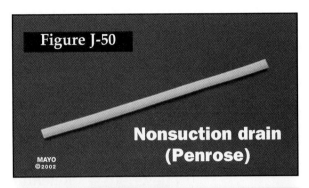

Figure J-50

Nonsuction drain (Penrose)

MAYO ©2002

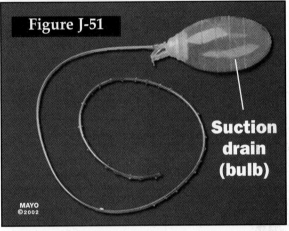

Figure J-51

Suction drain (bulb)

MAYO ©2002

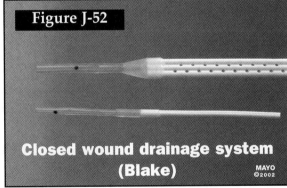

Figure J-52

Closed wound drainage system (Blake)

MAYO ©2002

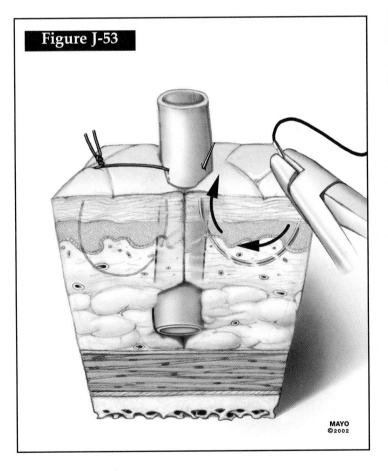

Figure J-53

MAYO ©2002

J. Wound Closure

9. Retention Suture (Bolster)

When there is a threat of wound rupture in abdominal surgery a retention suture (bolster) is used in the anterior abdominal wall **(Figure J-53)**.

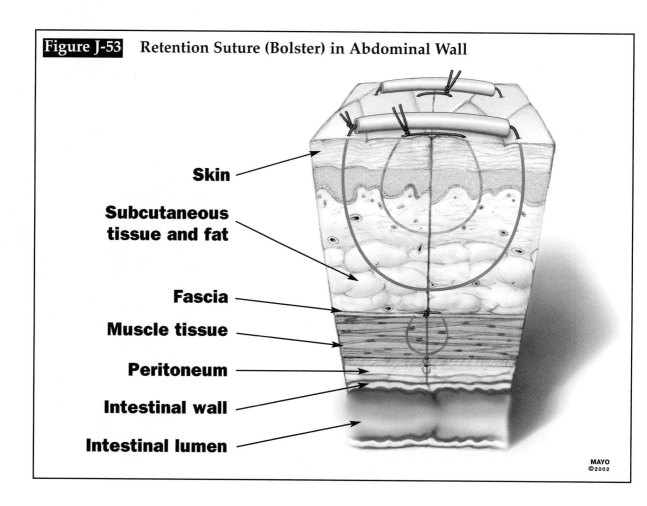

Figure J-53 Retention Suture (Bolster) in Abdominal Wall

Skin

Subcutaneous tissue and fat

Fascia

Muscle tissue

Peritoneum

Intestinal wall

Intestinal lumen

MAYO
©2002

J. Wound Closure

10. Closure of the Anterior Abdominal Wall

When closing the anterior abdominal wall it is critical that all anatomic layers be closed individually **(Figure J-53)**.

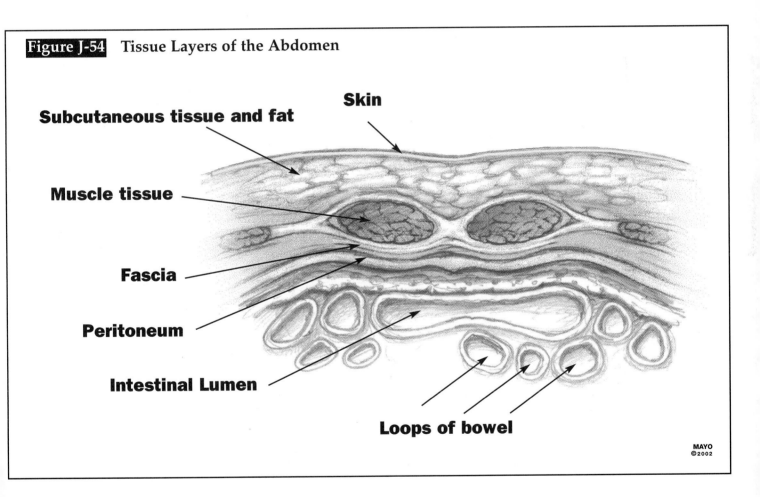

Figure J-54   Tissue Layers of the Abdomen

Skin

Subcutaneous tissue and fat

Muscle tissue

Fascia

Peritoneum

Intestinal Lumen

Loops of bowel

MAYO
©2002

J. Wound Closure

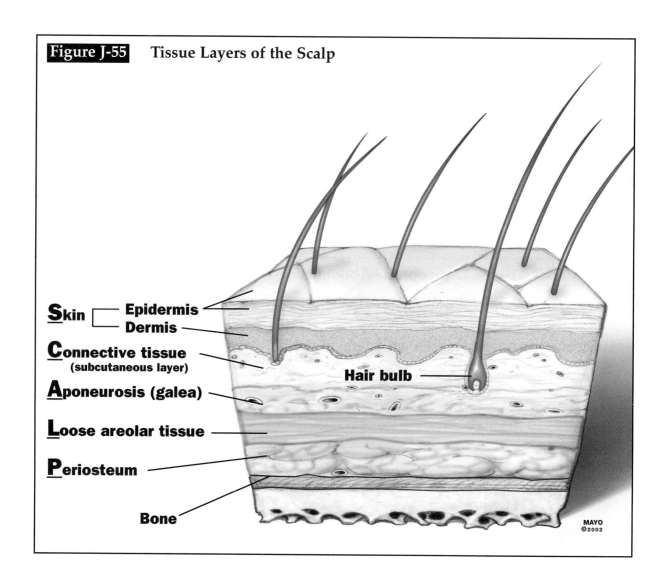

Figure J-55   Tissue Layers of the Scalp

Skin ⌐ **Epidermis**
     ⌐ **Dermis**

Connective tissue
(subcutaneous layer)

Aponeurosis (galea)

Loose areolar tissue

Periosteum

Bone

Hair bulb

MAYO
©2002

11. Closure of a Scalp Wound

When closing lacerations of the scalp it is critical that all anatomic layers be closed individually **(Figure J-55)**. If the laceration extends through the galea aponeurosis or deeper, then the galea should be closed with 2-0 or 3-0 absorbable sutures. Care is taken not to place sutures in the layer superficial to the galea which is the subcuataneous connective tissue layer in which the hair bulbs reside **(Figures J-55)**. If this connective tissue layer is closed scar alopecia (bald spot at the scar) can occur. The hair bearing skin is usually closed with surgical staples. If the laceration does not extend to the galea then only the skin is closed.

Quiz

Fill in the blank with the correct letter relating to suture method. Answers below.

1. ____
2. ____
3. ____
4. ____
5. ____
6. ____
7. ____
8. ____

A. Simple Interrupted
B. Vertical Mattress
C. Horizontal Mattress
D. Running (Baseball Stitch)
E. Running Lock
F. Running Intracuticular
G. Running Intracuticular with Loop
H. Purse String

1.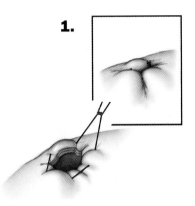

2.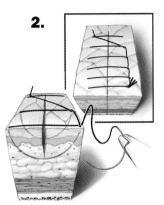

3.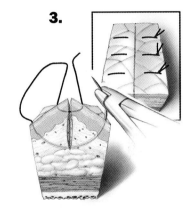

4.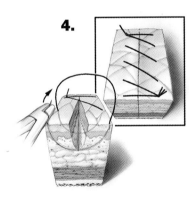

5.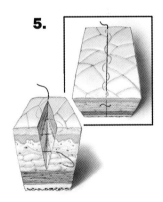

6.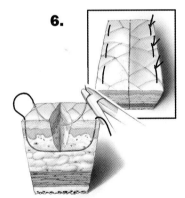

7.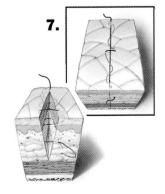

8.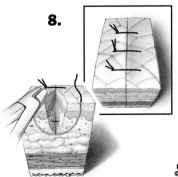

Answers

1. H	5. F
2. E	6. C
3. B	7. G
4. D	8. A

MAYO
©2002

K. Skin Flaps

1. Introduction

A piece of skin that has been excised (removed) for one reason or another (e.g., it contained a lesion) leaves a hole in the remaining skin. This hole can be closed by a skin flap so that healing can occur by primary intention. Skin flaps optimally close the defect without tension.

Care is taken to stay in the subcutaneous plane during excision of the lesion. Countertraction is helpful during incision and excision. The scissors can be used to undermine as well as cut the deep layers of the soft tissue. The skin incisions themselves should be made with a sharp knife. Incisions should be made perpendicular to the skin edges.

2. Fusiform (Elliptical) Excision

Fusiform excision is a simple way to excise skin lesions **(Figure K-1)**. An elliptical incision is made around the lesion, the length of which is 1.5 to 3 times the width of the lesion. If the width-to-length ratio is any closer to 1:1, then the wound will usually close with puckering at the ends. Once excised, the wound is undermined and closed by the principle of halving **(Figure K-2)**. The drawings **(Figure K-3)** show the technique of the fusiform incision **(Figure K-3A)**, excision **(Figure K-3B),** undermining **(Figure K-3C)**, and closure **(Figure K-3D).** The fusiform excision and undermining is a type of advancement flap which allows skin closure without tension.

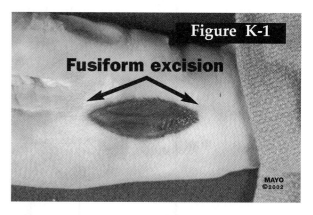

Figure K-1

Fusiform excision

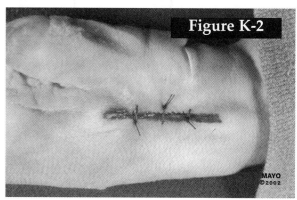

Figure K-2

178

K. Skin Flaps

FUSIFORM (ELIPTICAL) EXCISION

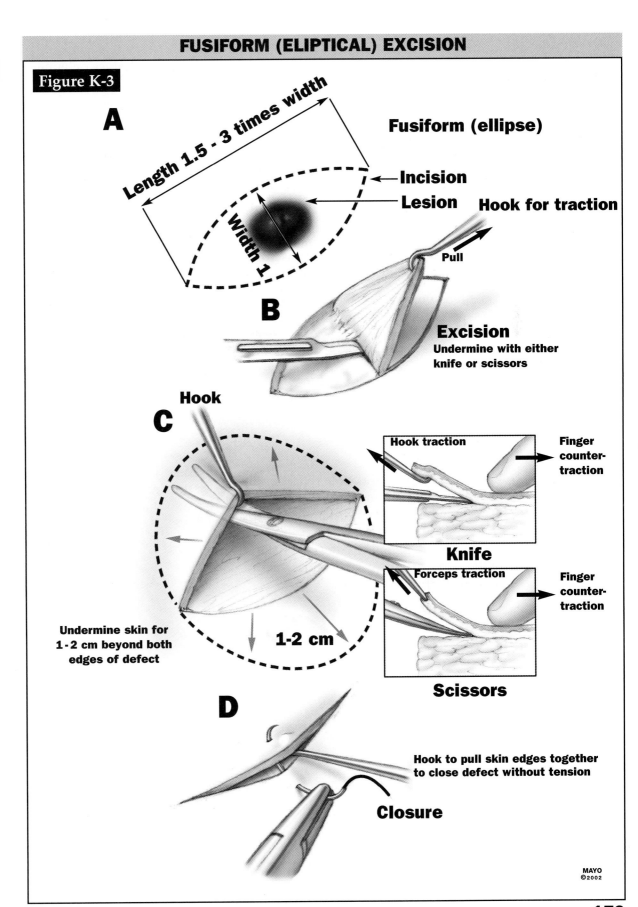

Figure K-3

A

Length 1.5 - 3 times width

Width 1

Fusiform (ellipse)

← Incision

Lesion

Hook for traction

Pull

B

Excision
Undermine with either
knife or scissors

C

Hook

Hook traction

Finger
counter-
traction

Knife

Forceps traction

Finger
counter-
traction

Scissors

Undermine skin for
1 - 2 cm beyond both
edges of defect

1-2 cm

D

Hook to pull skin edges together
to close defect without tension

Closure

K. Skin Flaps

3. Advancement Flap

The advancement flap is rectangular with a 2 to 3 length-to-width ratio **(Figure K-4)**. The skin defect is in the small shaded square, which is excised. After excision of the lesion, the two sides of the flap are incised and the entire flap is undermined in the layer between the skin and the deeper subcutaneous tissues. The skin adjacent to the long edges of the incision is also undermined for 1-2 centimeters to allow for increased flap mobility and wound closure without tension.

The first suture is placed in the center of the flap and is tied with a hand tie and a surgeon's knot **(Figure K-5)**. By keeping constant tension on the sutures, one can prevent tying an "air knot." The suture is cut with a 3 to 4 millimeter tail to prevent unwinding of the material over time. The corner stitches are placed next, as they are at the other sites of primary tension in this flap design **(Figure K-5)**.

Because of the excision, note that the skin edge is longer than the flap edge **(Figure K-5)**. These incisions are closed with the principle of halving. The next suture is placed in the middle of the lower edge of the flap and in the middle of the corresponding skin **(Figure K-6)**.

The two halves on either side of the lower edge are still uneven, but less so now. The next suture is placed between the halves of each of these segments according to the principle of halving. Subsequent sutures then split the difference between previous sutures until enough sutures are placed for an adequate closure of the lower edge **(Figure K-7)**. In this way the redundant skin of the lower edge is spread evenly across the entire wound closure and results in a smooth wound edge.

The upper edge is closed in an uneven manner, resulting in a standing cone or "dog ear" deformity **(Figure K-6)**. How do you fix a standing cone? First a back cut is made **(Figure K-6, K-7)**. The standing cone back cut **(Figure K-6, K-7)** is always done away from the flap pedicle. The excess skin is excised **(Figure K-8)**. After the triangle of excess skin is trimmed the flap is inset to give a good fit **(Figure K-9)**. The flap is then sutured into place and the standing cone deformity is resolved. **Figure K-10** shows the final advancement flap along with the skin that was excised.

K. Skin Flaps

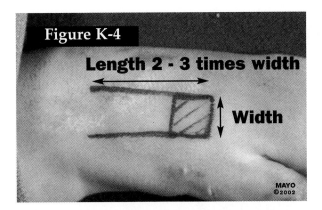

Figure K-4

Length 2 - 3 times width

Width

MAYO
©2002

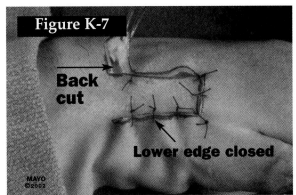

Figure K-7

Back cut

Lower edge closed

MAYO
©2002

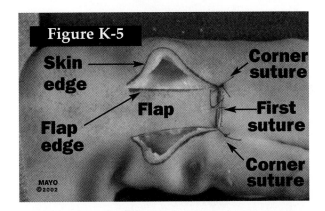

Figure K-5

Skin edge

Corner suture

Flap

First suture

Flap edge

Corner suture

MAYO
©2002

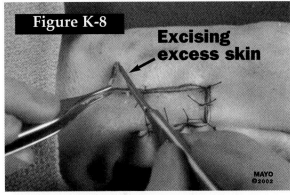

Figure K-8

Excising excess skin

MAYO
©2002

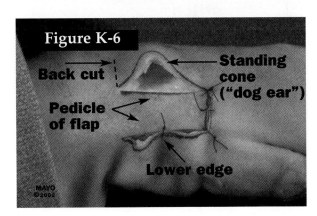

Figure K-6

Back cut

Standing cone ("dog ear")

Pedicle of flap

Lower edge

MAYO
©2002

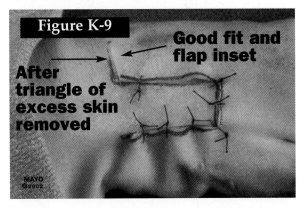

Figure K-9

Good fit and flap inset

After triangle of excess skin removed

MAYO
©2002

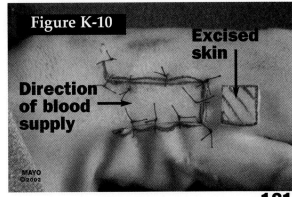

Figure K-10

Excised skin

Direction of blood supply

MAYO
©2002

K. Skin Flaps

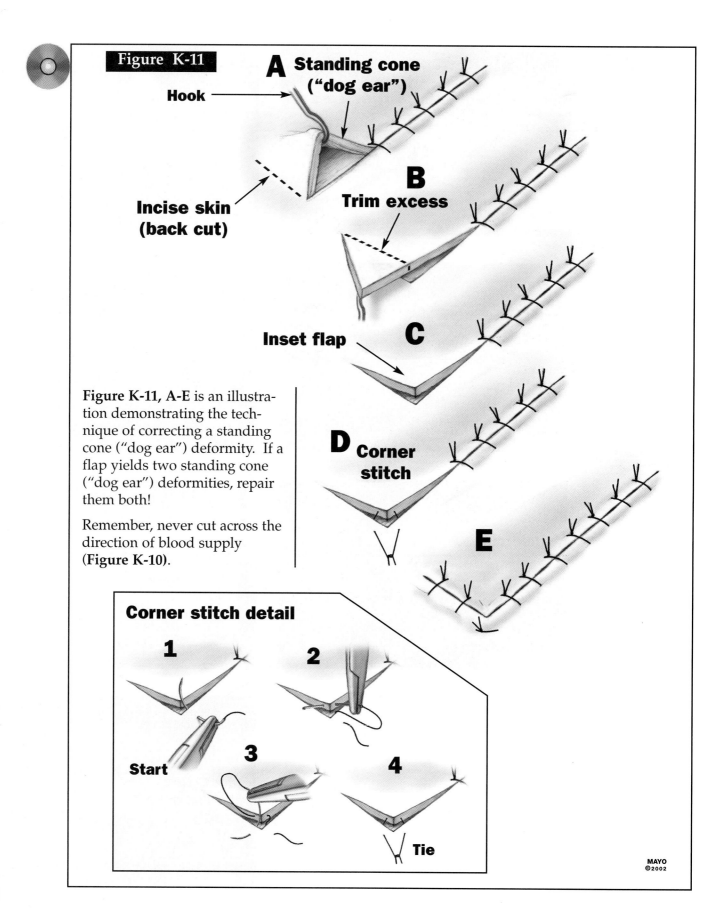

Figure K-11

A Standing cone ("dog ear")

Hook

Incise skin (back cut)

B Trim excess

C Inset flap

D Corner stitch

E

Figure K-11, A-E is an illustration demonstrating the technique of correcting a standing cone ("dog ear") deformity. If a flap yields two standing cone ("dog ear") deformities, repair them both!

Remember, never cut across the direction of blood supply (**Figure K-10**).

Corner stitch detail

1

2

Start

3

4

Tie

Quiz

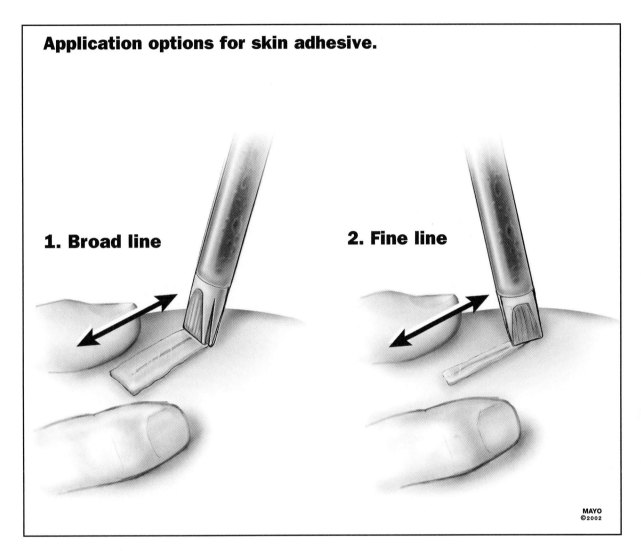

Application options for skin adhesive.

1. Broad line

2. Fine line

MAYO
©2002

Select and circle the method for closing a low tension skin wound with a skin adhesive. Circle the best choice A or B.

A. *Use 3 thin applications of skin adhesive 30 seconds apart for a low tension wound.*

B. *Use 2 thin applications of skin adhesive 30 seconds apart for a low tension wound.*

Answer

A

K. Skin Flaps

4 Rotation Flap

The rotation flap is utilized to close a triangular defect. The rotation flap follows a smooth curve from the site of the defect. It then gets rotated into place. Typically, the limb (arc) of rotation is 2-4 times longer than the limb (arc) of the defect it needs to close **(Figure K-12)**. This is a flap with a wide vascular pedicle and is extremely useful in facial reconstruction **(Figure K-13)**.

After the lesion is excised producing a triangular defect, the flap is incised with a knife and broadly undermined. A 1-2 centimeter margin around the skin edges of the defect is also undermined. The point of maximal rotation is also the point of maximal tension in this flap and it is inset first with a suture **(Figure K-13)**. The shorter flap edge is then closed to the longer skin edge with the principle of halving, splitting each side in half for subsequent suture placement. The rotation flap after closure, along with the excised triangular cutaneous defect, is shown in **Figure K-14**.

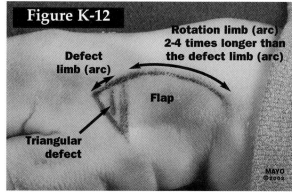

Figure K-12

Rotation limb (arc) 2-4 times longer than the defect limb (arc)

Defect limb (arc)

Flap

Triangular defect

Rotation limb (arc) is 2-4 times longer than triangular defect limb (arc).

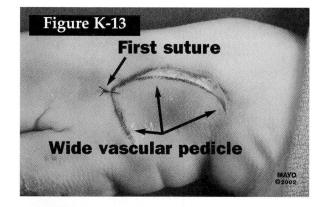

Figure K-13

First suture

Wide vascular pedicle

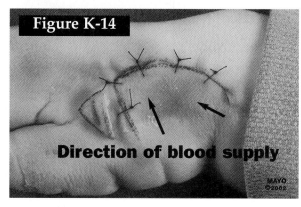

Figure K-14

Direction of blood supply

K. Skin Flaps

5. Z-plasty

The Z-plasty is useful in lengthening contracted scars to improve function as well as reorienting the direction of scars to improve cosmetic appearance. In this example **(Figure K-15)** the central limb **(line A to B)** is 3 cm at the start of the incision and would represent the scar to be excised and the axis that we want to lengthen **(Figure K-15)**. The upper flap, A, is stippled to show how it is transposed. This carries the central limb from a horizontal plane to a vertical plane **(Figures K-16)**. The limbs are the same length and both come off at the same angle from the central limb. The angle varies anywhere between 30° and 60°. The greater the angle, the greater the gain in wound length. Any sharper (smaller) angle results in risk of necrosis in the tip of the flap, while any broader angle results in a difficult rotation. Off any scar the limbs can be drawn in two different directions. Always draw the limbs more parallel to relaxed skin tension lines to result in the best scar result.

Both triangular flaps **(A and B, Figure K-16)** rotate opposite each other. Broad undermining is done under both flaps, as well as under the entire incised region, to allow ease of flap elevation and rotation. Each flap is then grasped with a forceps and transposed across so that the central limb totally reorients by 90° in this example **(Figure K-16)** from a central limb B-A **(Figure K-15)** to a new central limb at 1-2 **(Figure K-16)**. The width of the defect **increased** from 3cm to 4cm **(Figure K-15, see ruler)**, thus demonstrating the lengthening effect of a Z-plasty **(Figure K-17)**. The corner stitches are placed into each flap, **(Flap A and B at 1 and 2, Figure K-17)** first to transpose them. Always remember to transpose the Z-plasty. If it is closed as it was initially incised, it will have no effect!

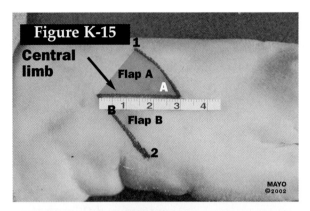

Figure K-15

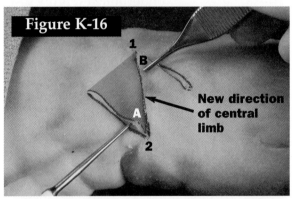

Figure K-16

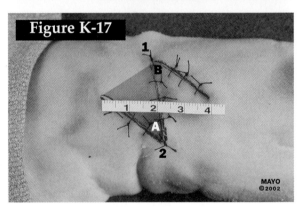

Figure K-17

K. Skin Flaps

6. Note Flap

The note flap is shaped like a musical note **(Figure K-18A)** and is designed to close a circular defect. The flap typically measures one and one half times the length of the diameter of the circular excision. A second line of the flap is then dropped at a 60° angle and is typically about the length of the diameter of the defect **(Figure K-18A)**. After the flap is incised, the wound and the flap are widely undermined **(Figure K-18B)**. The two triangular shaped flaps that result from this dissection are then transposed. Both triangular flaps rotate opposite each other. The triangular flap **(Flap X, Figure K-18B)** elevated adjacent to the defect is typically transposed and inset into the donor site **(Flap X to X')** with the first stitch **(Figure K-18C)** while flap Y is rotated to cover the site where the lesion was excised **(Figure K-18C)**. Care must be taken to deliver the flap Y out from under the flap X closure. The second flap **(flap Y)** is then inset with one suture to the lateral aspect of the defect. Here the suture is intentionally not placed at the point of the flap Y as the point will be trimmed and inset later **(Figure K-18D)**. The sites between are then closed by the principle of halving.

Commonly a "dog-ear" (standing cone) will ensue on the lateral aspect of the flap Y as it insets into the lateral (circular) defect **(Figure K-18E)**. After inset of the entire flap and the pointed corner has been trimmed carefully to improve the inset **(Figure K-18D)**, then the "dog-ear" can be addressed appropriately. To excise the "dog ear" a skin hook is placed at the apex of the puckered skin **(Figure K-18E)**. A site is marked away from the pedicle of the flap and a backcut is made **(Figure K-18E)**. The triangular portion of skin is undermined and the excess trimmed **(Figure K-18F)**. It is then inset and closed with simple sutures **(Figure K-18G,H)**.

K. Skin Flaps

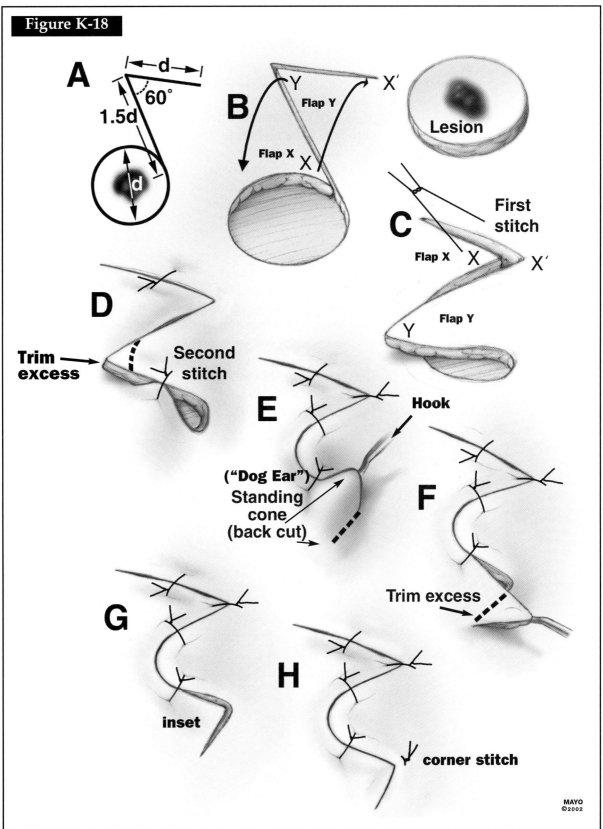

Figure K-18

A
d
60°
1.5d
d

B
Y
X′
Flap Y
Flap X
X

Lesion

C
First stitch
Flap X
X
X′
Flap Y
Y

D
Trim excess
Second stitch

E
Hook
("Dog Ear")
Standing cone (back cut)

F
Trim excess

G
inset

H
corner stitch

MAYO
©2002

187

K. Skin Flaps

7. Bilobe Flap

The bilobe flap is a dual transposition flap used to close circular defects. The diameter of the circular defect determines the size and shape of the other limbs **(Figure K-19 A-C)**. The diameter of the first limb is typically three-fourths to the same diameter as the defect and the diameter of the second limb is typically one-half to three-fourths the diameter of the original defect. The limbs will typically rotate 45° to 50° each. Any greater arc of rotation results in too much puckering and "dog-ear" formation. As shown in the diagram a small triangle adjacent to both the defect and the first limb at the inferior aspect of the circular defect needs to be excised to facilitate rotation of the first limb into the defect **(Figure K-19 A-C)**. The length from the defect margin to the point where the triangle to be excised reaches its peak (pivot point, **Figure K-19A)** is typically one-half the diameter of the defect, or in other words, the radius of the defect. This triangle to be excised can vary depending on the specific tissues.

Once the lesion is excised, the triangular tissue is excised, and everything is undermined, the first limb is rotated into place. Typically, the first suture is placed at the peak between the first and second limb of this bilobe flap or at a more lateral aspect on the defect to pull the first limb into the defect site **(Figure K-19C-D)**. Care is taken to tie this down well. Now you can see limb 1 and limb 2 are rotated and X lines up withX', Y lines up with Y', and Z lines up with Z' **(Figure K-19D)**. The order of the stitches placed is not as critical as putting the stitches in accurately to facilitate closure. Again, like the note flap, in this bilobe flap there is one triangular shaped limb of the flap being inset into a circular defect. Limb 2 is cut into a more triangular shape **(Figure K-19C)** in order to facilitate the donor site closure as a linear scar. This triangular tip of limb 2 usually has to be trimmed for proper inset of the flap **(Figure K-19E)**. Once the other limbs are closed the pointed tip of limb 2 is then trimmed off. The rest of the wound is then closed with simple sutures **(Figure K-19 A-F)**.

BILOBE FLAP

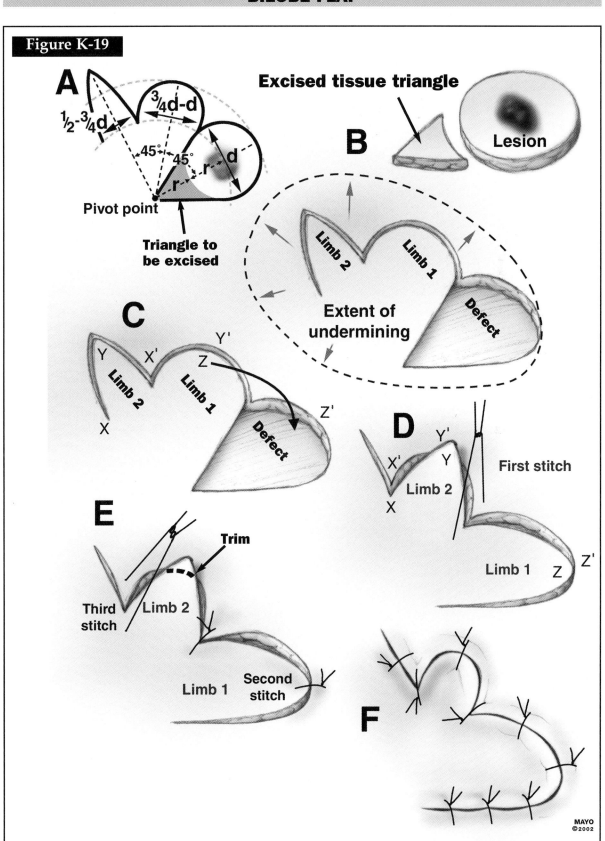

Figure K-19

A
½-¾d
¾d-d
45° 45°
r r d
Pivot point
Triangle to be excised

B
Excised tissue triangle
Lesion
Limb 2
Limb 1
Defect
Extent of undermining

C
Y X'
Y'
Z
Limb 2
Limb 1
Defect
X
Z'

D
Y'
X' Y
First stitch
Limb 2
X
Limb 1
Z Z'

E
Trim
Third stitch
Limb 2
Limb 1
Second stitch

F

MAYO
©2002

189

K. Skin Flaps

8. Rhombic Flap

The rhombic or rhomboid flap is designed as a parallelogram with the wide angles of about 120° and the narrow angles at about 60°. All sides of the parallelogram (diamond) to be excised **(Figure K-20,A-B)** are the same length as is the length of each limb of the flap. The limb coming off of the parallelogram **(Figure K-20A, line B-B′)** is on a line continued as a connection of the 120° angles. The limb **(Figure K-20A, line B′-C)** is then dropped up or down from there and parallel to the lateral wall of the parallelogram. The lesion is excised in the shape of a diamond (parallelogram) and the flap is incised and dissected with wide undermining. The point of maximal tension is the point where the apex of the flap limb meets the parallelogram **(Figure K-20, C at X-X′)**. In this case, the first point of the parallelogram is used as the site for the first suture **(Figure K-20, C at X-X′)**. Subsequent sutures are then placed to close each point of the flap **(Figure K-20 C-E)**. Deep sutures are used as needed. The angles of the parallelogram can vary. The side lengths can also vary in more complex reconstructions. After the lesion is removed, the closure is shown in the last drawing **(Figure K-20E)**.

K. Skin Flaps

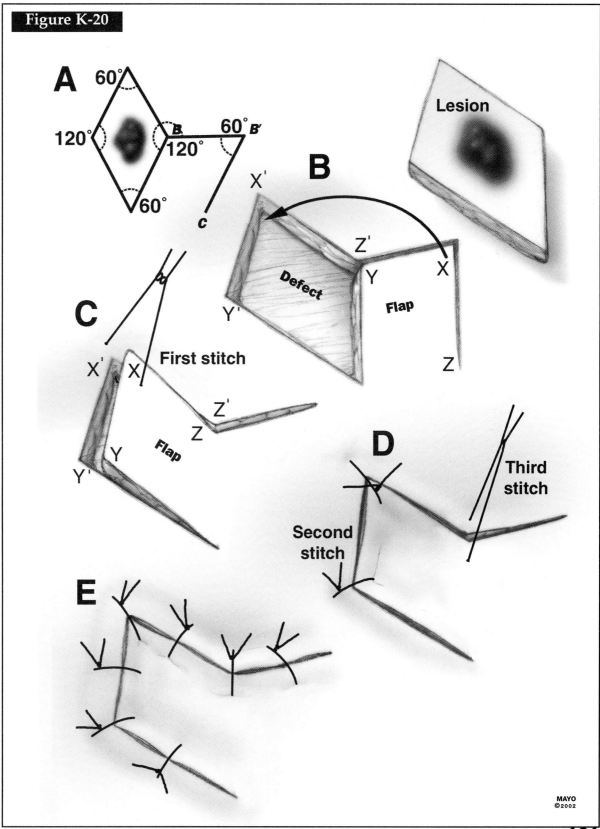

Figure K-20

L. Scar Excision and Closure

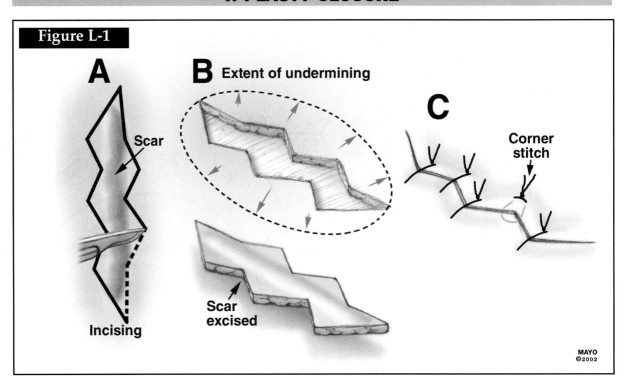

Figure L-1

A

Scar

Incising

B Extent of undermining

Scar excised

C

Corner stitch

MAYO
©2002

1. W-plasty Closure

The W-plasty is a simple way to change a scar into a more angulated shape. This break in the continuity of the scar makes it less likely that the viewing eye will follow the entire length of the angulated line; thereby tending to camoflage the scar which makes it less perceptible. In humans the limbs of the W-plasty are typically about 5 to 7 millimeters long. The W- plasty has two sides that are mirror images of each other. It is imperative in this type of scar revision to make sure that each peak on one side corresponds to the valley on the opposite side. If not, excision and subsequent closure will be difficult. After the scar is excised, wide undermining is performed around the site of the peaks and valleys. Peaks and valleys are closed to each other with sutures **(Figure L-1, A-C)**. Subsequent sutures along the limbs can be placed as needed. Corner stitches may or may not be used at the peak valley contacts. Again, palpation by pressing the wound

*The W-plasty scar revision technique camouflages scars **not parallel** to relaxed skin tension lines (RSTL). By breaking up a scar from linear to irregular, the eye does not follow it as well, and the scar is less apparent. The opposite sides of the scar excision are mirror images of each other so that each peak corresponds to a valley on the opposite side. The limbs of the W-plasty should not typically be longer than 5 to 7millimeters. The angles should not be less than 90°. Deep sutures are placed as needed. The skin sutures should be placed at each peak **(Figure L-1 A-C)**.*

together intermittently allows the operator to see if enough undermining has been done to facilitate wound closure. The angles of the W-plasties are about 90° degrees to each, athough they can vary. They should not be greater than 90° or the camouflaging result is not as good.

L. Scar Excision and Closure

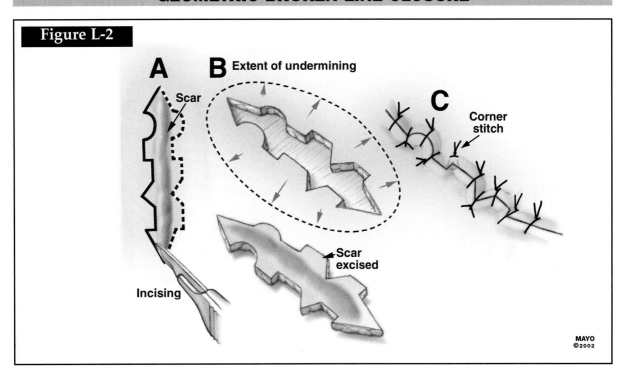

Figure L-2

A B Extent of undermining

Scar

Incising

C

Corner stitch

Scar excised

MAYO
©2002

2. Geometric Broken Line Closure

Geometric broken line closure is used to break up linear scars into irregular shapes. This is based on the premise that the eye has a difficult time following broken lines and this makes the scar less perceptible. With the geometric broken line closure, each side is drawn as a mirror image of the opposite side. On the face, the limbs typically will not be greater than 5 to 7 millimeters long. After excision of the scar the wound is widely undermined in all directions. Care is taken to do the closure meticulously. Subcutaneous sutures are used as necessary. By pushing on the soft tissue it is possible to get an idea whether the undermining has been adequate enough to allow a tension free closure. In scar revision on humans it is best to use long lasting absorbable sutures in the deep layers to facilitate tensile strength building in the wound. A corner stitch can be used at any site where a corner is brought together. In this example a corner stitch is placed into one of the 90° peaks for demonstration pur-

*Geometric broken line closure is useful on long hypertrophic scars **nearly parallel** to relaxed skin tension lines (RSTL), but not tethered. The irregular border makes the scar less apparent, as the eye follows straight lines well, but not broken lines. Like the W-plasty, each side is a mirror image of the opposite side. It is even more irregular a border than a W-plasty. Sutures are placed to close the wound using the principle of halving* **(Figure L-2, A-C)**.

poses. Sometimes simple sutures placed into corners will result in inversion of the corner and result in a less acceptable scar. Corner stitches do not necessarily have to be placed at every corner closure. After a scar is revised using the geometric broken line closure dermabrasion may be used at a later date to further improve the scar.

193

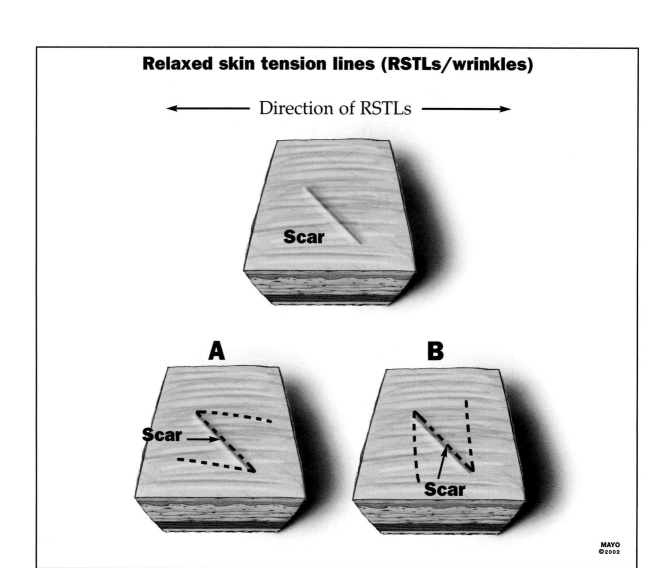

Relaxed skin tension lines (RSTLs/wrinkles)

← Direction of RSTLs →

Scar

A

Scar →

B

Scar

MAYO
©2002

The scar is to be excised and reoriented. In both A and B the scar is in the same direction in relation to the relaxed skin tension lines (RSTLs). The RSTLs are identified by the wrinkles. Which Z-plasty design will result in a better scar after flap transposition? Example A or B? Circle your choice.

Answer

A

Quiz

Fill in the shaded blanks! See page 182, Figure K-11 for the correct answers.

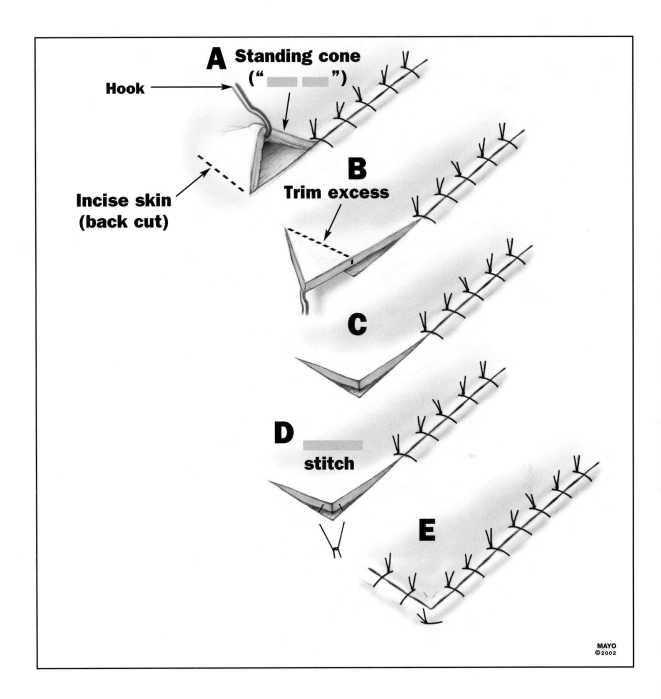

A Standing cone
("⬚⬚ ⬚⬚")

Hook →

Incise skin
(back cut)

B Trim excess

C

D ⬚⬚ stitch

E

MAYO
©2002

M. Postoperative Wound Care

1. Local Wound Care

In general it is best to keep the wound dry during healing. Avoid allowing excessive moisture in and around the wound. It may be helpful for the patient to clean the wound with alcohol or hydrogen peroxide to remove blood, debris and "crusts" of dried blood. Antibiotic ointment may be placed on the sutures two or three times a day to keep them from getting crusted.

It is usually safe to bathe by the second or third day after surgery and it may be necessary to cover the wound with a piece of plastic. On postoperative visits, re-examine the wound, especially if the patient complains of pain or tenderness. Observe the wound for swelling, redness (**erythema**), tenderness to palpation, and drainage from the wound. The patient may also experience fear. Be kind. If any of these findings occur, it may be necessary to reopen the wound to make sure that an abscess is not forming.

2. Suture Removal

The time for suture removal depends upon the location of the wound, but in the facial region, it usually ranges from the fifth to the seventh postoperative day. It is usually best to pick up the knotted end of the suture with a fine forceps. A suture-removal scissors is then applied to cut the suture and remove it as atraumatically as possible. On occasion, it may be necessary, after sutures have been removed, to then apply steri-strips to help support the wound, especially if removal is on or about the fifth day.

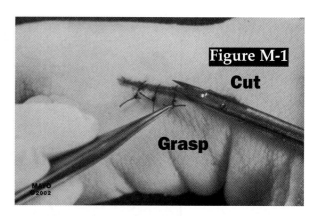

Figure M-1
Cut
Grasp

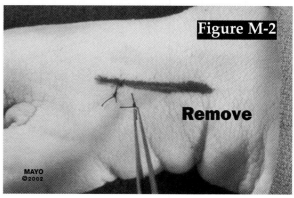

Figure M-2
Remove

a. Simple Suture Removal

Note how in **Figure M-1,** the knotted end is grasped with the pickup forceps, and the distal end is cut adjacent to the skin. **Figure M-2** demonstrates the removal of the simple suture so that the edge of the suture is not dragged through the wound. Be sure **not to cut** the sutures in 2 spots; otherwise, you have nothing to pull the suture through the wound! You do not want to leave a permanent suture in the skin wound.

M. Postoperative Wound Care

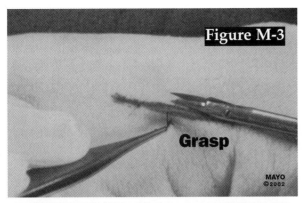

Figure M-3

Grasp

MAYO
©2002

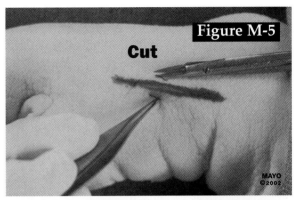

Figure M-5

Cut

MAYO
©2002

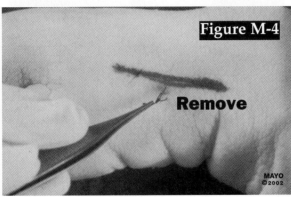

Figure M-4

Remove

MAYO
©2002

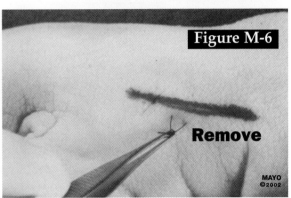

Figure M-6

Remove

MAYO
©2002

b. Vertical Mattress Suture Removal
Grasp the knotted end with a fine forceps and cut the looped end with the fine suture scissors **(Figure M-3)**. **Figure M-4** demonstrates the removal of the suture.

c. Horizontal Mattress Suture Removal
Grasp the knotted end and cut the suture on the opposite side to remove the suture atraumatically **(Figures M-5,6)**.

M. Postoperative Wound Care

d. Simple Running Suture ("Baseball Stitch") Removal

Grasp one knotted end and use the suture scissors to cut the looped end **(Figure M-7)**. Continue cutting the looped ends **(Figure M-8)**. Once you reach the other knotted end at the extreme end of the wound, remove each loop just as if you were removing simple sutures **(Figure M-9)**.

e. Running-lock Suture Removal

Again, start at one end, grasping the knot, and use a fine suture scissors to cut the loop **(Figure M-10)**. Proceed down the wound, cutting the locked loops as you continue down to the end of the suture line **(Figure M-11)**. Then remove each suture individually as if you were removing a simple suture **(Figure M-12)**.

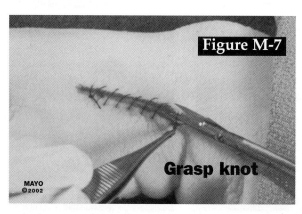

Figure M-7 — Grasp knot

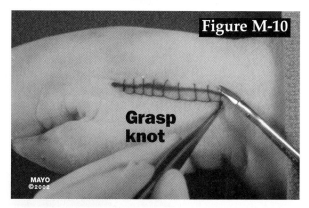

Figure M-10 — Grasp knot

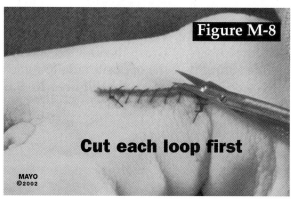

Figure M-8 — Cut each loop first

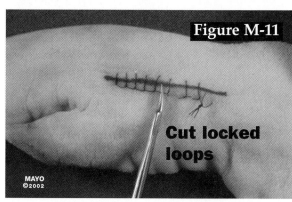

Figure M-11 — Cut locked loops

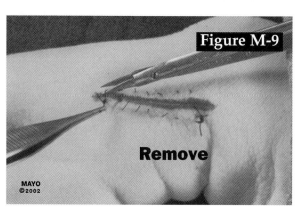

Figure M-9 — Remove

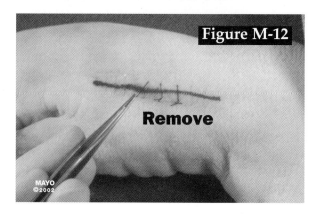

Figure M-12 — Remove

M. Postoperative Wound Care

f. Running Intracuticular Suture Removal

Cut the suture loop in the midportion of the wound **(Figure M-13)**. Extract the suture on the left side of the wound by pulling on the suture with a forceps **(Figure M-14)**. Then pull and extract the suture on the right side of the wound with a forceps **(Figure M-15)**.

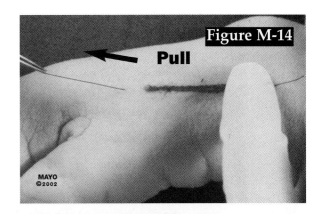

Figure M-14

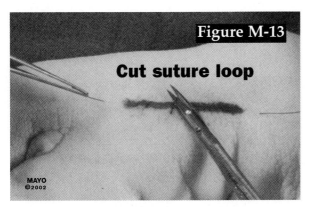

Figure M-13

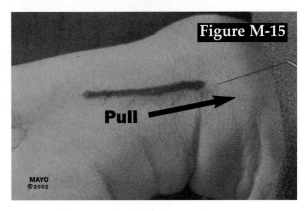

Figure M-15

M. Postoperative Wound Care

3. Staple Removal

Pick up the staple removal instrument and approach the wound along its long axis **(Figure M-16)**. Then engage the staple removal instrument beneath the staple **(Figure M-17).** Close the staple removal instrument and extract the staple **(Figure M-18)**. Continue until all the staples are removed **(Figure M-19)**. On occasion, it may be necessary to use steri-strips to help keep small portions of the wound which have **dehisced** (come apart) in proper position.

4. Drain Removal

Most drains are sutured in place with a simple suture. All that is necessary is to cut the suture with the suture scissors. Grasp the knotted end with the forceps and remove the suture. Once the suture is removed the drain will be free to be shortened, cut, or completely extracted. Suction drains should be removed from suction prior to removal.

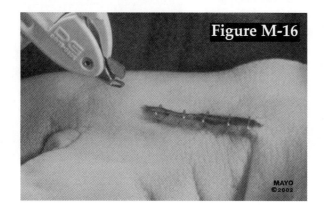

Figure M-16

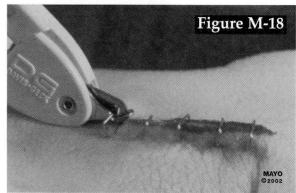

Figure M-18

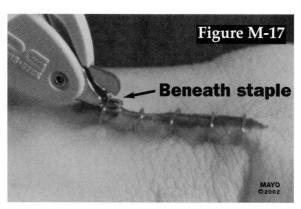

Figure M-17

← **Beneath staple**

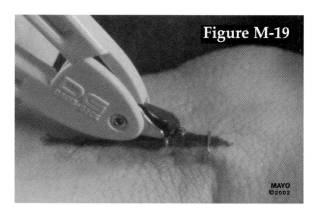

Figure M-19

Quiz

Fill in the blank! See below for the correct answers.

Table H-1 Increasing tensile strength of the wound after injury

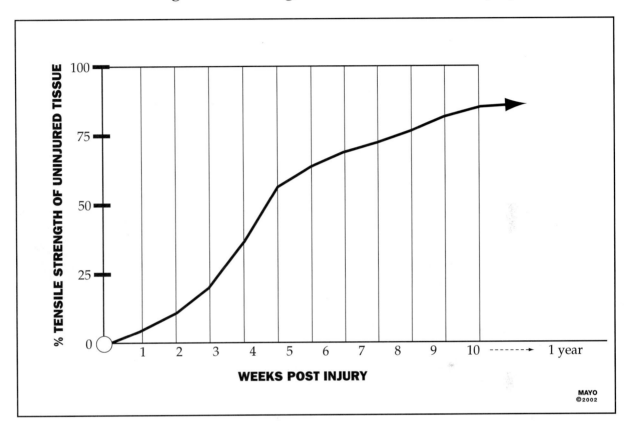

Tensile strength of a healing wound is never better than _____ of uninjured tissue.

Answer _____

%08

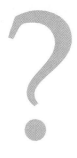

N. 100 Quiz Questions

How about a test of your knowledge? If you cannot answer a question, just move on to the next question. The answers are provided on page 212. No peeking! Circle the best choice before checking the answers.

1. Which blood cells are most intimately involved in the hemostatic process:
   a. Erythrocytes.
   b. Lymphocytes.
   c. Platelets.
   d. All of the above.
   e. None of above.

2. Control of major vascular bleeding both arterial or venous usually requires:
   a. Hemostatic clamps and ligature.
   b. Cautery and figure of 8 suture.
   c. Bone wax with fibrin glue.
   d. Bone wax with major thrombin.
   e. None of the above.

3. Major options to control intraoperative bleeding and obtain hemostasis are:
   a. Digital pressure.
   b. A tourniquet.
   c. Hemostatic clamps.
   d. Two of the above.
   e. None of the above.

4. The primary disadvantage of cautery to obtain surgical hemostasis is the:
   a. High cost.
   b. Potential for severe tissue damage which can delay wound healing.
   c. Inability to control minor bleeding.
   d. Need for extensive training in the use of the device(s).
   e. None of the above.

5. This substance breaks down fibrinogen and may be sprayed onto surfaces to inhibit bleeding:
   a. Thrombin.
   b. Epinephrine.
   c. Avitene S.
   d. Gelatin.
   e. None of the above.

6. Fibrin glue is a mixture of:
   a. Fibrinogen and thrombin.
   b. Plasminogen and thrombin.
   c. Fibrinogen and fibrin.
   d. Plasminogen and fibrin.
   e. Two of the above.

7. Topical hemostats can be used alone to control arterial bleeding
   a. True.
   b. False.
   c. Always.
   d. Two of the above.
   e. None of the above.

8. The type of topical hemostat that provides the fastest hemostasis is:
   a. A gelatin sponge.
   b. Topical thrombin (USP Thrombinogen).
   c. A fibrin glue.
   d. A collagen pad.
   e. None of the above.

9. Seven days after suturing, tensile strength of a wound will be:
   a. 5% of uninjured tissue.
   b. 20% of uninjured tissue.
   c. 30% of uninjured tissue.
   d. 40% of uninjured tissue.
   e. 50% of uninjured tissue.

10. In a completely healed wound, the tensile strength will be:
    a. 20% of uninjured tissue.
    b. 40% of uninjured tissue.
    c. 60% of uninjured tissue.
    d. 80% of uninjured tissue.
    e. Just about (90+ %) back to normal.

11. An anesthesiologist is:
    a. a surgeon
    b. a physician specializing in administration of anesthetics
    c. a physician specializing in the lung
    d. a physician specializing in the gastrointestinal tract
    e. none of the above

12. Bacteremia is:
    a. an infection
    b. bacteria in the gastrointestinal tract
    c. the presence of bacteria in the blood
    d. the presence of bacteria in the urine
    e. none of the above

13. Cardiopulmonary pertains to:
    a. the heart and lungs
    b. the heart
    c. the lungs
    d. the kidney
    e. all of the above

14. Cellulitis is:
    a. inflammation of cells
    b. inflammation of fat
    c. inflammation of the brain
    d. inflammation of muscle
    e. none of the above

N. 100 Quiz Questions

15. Cicatrix is:
    a. a scar
    b. a wound
    c. a part of the kidney
    d. a part of bone
    e. all of the above

16. Collagen is:
    a. a blood-borne substance
    b. a substance present in neurologic tissue
    c. the protein substance of connective tissues
    d. the mineralized matrix of bone
    e. all of the above

17. Debridement is:
    a. the process of making an incision
    b. the removal of foreign material or dead tissue
    c. the laying down of bone by osteoblasts
    d. the process of obtaining hemostasis
    e. none of the above

18. Dehiscence is:
    a. the removal of foreign material
    b. the act of removing diseased tissue
    c. the separation of the layers of a surgical wound
    d. the falling apart of a wound
    e. both c and d

19. Devitalized is:
    a. to deprive of vitality or of life
    b. the removal of internal organs
    c. the death of tissue
    d. all of the above
    e. a and c

20. An electrolyte is:
    a. sodium
    b. chloride
    c. substance that dissociates-associates into ions when in solution
    d. potassium
    e. all of the above

21. "Endocrine" means:
    a. pertaining to internal secretion of a hormonal nature
    b. pertaining to blood-borne bacteria
    c. pertaining to the elements of blood
    d. pertaining to neurologic tissue
    e. none of the above

22. "Enzyme" means:
    a. a substance that is changed during a chemical reaction
    b. a protein molecule that participates in a chemical reaction by speeding the chemical reaction
    c. a carbohydrate moiety that speeds chemical reactions
    d. none of the above
    e. all of the above

23. Epinephrine is:
    a. a primary constituent of bone
    b. a drug used to open clogged blood vessels
    c. a vasoconstrictive agent that causes blood vessels to narrow or shrink down
    d. none of the above
    e. all of the above

24. "Erythematous" means:
    a. whiteness of the skin
    b. redness of the skin
    c. loss of vascular supply to the skin
    d. dullness of the skin
    e. loss of tissue oxygenation

25. Fibroblasts are:
    a. a red blood cell
    b. a kidney cell
    c. a cardiac muscle cell
    d. a smooth muscle cell
    e. a connective-tissue cell producing collagen

26. Gangrene is:
    a. loss of kidney function
    b. loss of the ability of the lungs to work adequately
    c. death of tissue secondary to trauma
    d. death of tissue due to a loss of vascular supply followed by infection
    e. none of the above

27. The formation in wounds of fleshy masses, which include a large amount of new blood vessels, during the healing process is:
    a. angiogenesis
    b. scar
    c. gangrene
    d. granulation tissue
    e. none of the above

28. A collection of blood in an organ or tissue due to a break in the wall of the blood vessel is:
    a. a hematoma
    b. the swollen space that contains blood

c. an abscess
d. all of the above
e. a and b

29. The interruption of the flow of blood through any vessel to any anatomical area is known as:
    a. cellulitis
    b. dehiscence
    c. erythema
    d. keloid
    e. hemostasis

30. HIV stands for:
    a. the human immunodeficiency virus
    b. the virus that causes AIDS (acquired immunodeficiency syndrome)
    c. hepatic immunodeficiency virus
    d. all of the above
    e. a and b

31. The overgrowth of scar tissue is known as:
    a. osteogenesis scar
    b. geographic scar
    c. tumor-like scar
    d. devitalization cicatrix
    e. hypertrophic scar

32. The body system that protects against infection and infectious disease is known as:
    a. the endocrine system
    b. the musculoskeletal system
    c. the pulmonary system
    d. the collagen system
    e. none of the above

33. The body's protective response caused by injury or destruction of tissue is known as:
    a. inflammation
    b. angiogenesis
    c. embryogenesis
    d. reflex
    e. symptomatology

34. Intubation is:
    a. the placement of a tube into a body canal or hollow organ
    b. the placement of a tube into the trachea
    c. the placement of a tube into the stomach
    d. all of the above
    e. none of the above

35. Keloids are:
    a. broken bones
    b. renal cells
    c. the end result of all scarring
    d. enlarged scar due to formation of excessive amounts of collagen
    e. enlarged scar due to formation of excessive amounts of cartilage

36. Lymphocytes are:
    a. red blood cells found in the blood, lymph, and lymphoid tissues
    b. white blood cells found in the blood, lymph, and lymphoid tissues
    c. tumor cells
    d. cells which reproduce in an uncontrolled manner by sexual reproduction
    e. none of the above

37. The sum of all the physical and chemical processes by which living organisms maintain their function and survive is known as:
    a. metaphysical functions
    b. holistic functions
    c. metabolic functions
    d. biochemical functions
    e. anabolic functions

38. A nurse trained in the administration of anesthetics is known as:
    a. an anesthesiologist
    b. a somnologist
    c. a nurse anesthetist
    d. an oncologist
    e. none of the above

39. The branch of medicine which studies basic elements of disease, especially changes in the body caused by disease, is:
    a. ophthalmology
    b. biochemistry
    c. oncology
    d. otorhinolaryngology
    e. pathology

40. "Perioperative" pertains to:
    a. the time period just before surgery
    b. the time period from the time of surgery to the time of discharge from the hospital
    c. the time period from one day prior to one day post-surgery
    d. two of the above
    e. all of the above

41. The time period occurring after a surgical operation is known as:
    a. postoperative
    b. perioperative
    c. operative
    d. two of the above
    e. all of the above

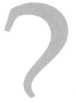

42. A seroma is also known as:
    a. a hematoma
    b. a chyloma
    c. a collection of serum in the tissues
    d. a serous cell tumor
    e. two of the above

43. Serum is:
    a. a body fluid consisting of vascular fluid devoid of white blood cells
    b. a body fluid consisting of vascular fluid devoid of white blood cells and platelets
    c. a body fluid consisting of vascular fluid devoid of red blood cells
    d. a body fluid consisting of vascular fluid devoid of platelets
    e. none of the above

44. The branch of medicine which treats diseases, injuries, and deformities by operation is:
    a. psychiatry
    b. internal medicine
    c. obstetrics
    d. pediatrics
    e. surgery

45. The term vasoconstrictive describes:
    a. a diminished caliber of blood vessels
    b. the loss of fatty tissues
    c. to narrow or shrink down blood vessels
    d. all of the above
    e. a and c

46. Viscera describes:
    a. the internal organs located inside the body cavity
    b. the renal system
    c. the hematopoietic system
    d. the musculoskeletal system
    e. the neurologic system

47. Tissue layers include:
    a. skin
    b. subcutaneous tissue
    c. fascia
    d. periosteum
    e. all of the above

48. The removal of damaged and dead tissue in a wound occurs during:
    a. the inflammation stage
    b. the proliferation of scar formation stage
    c. the scar maturation stage
    d. all of the above
    e. none of the above

49. Scar maturation:
    a. occurs immediately following the inflammatory stage
    b. occurs on days 5-14 and consists of the initiation of production of collagen fibers
    d. is not a distinct phase of wounding
    e. has a variable duration depending upon the specific type of tissues that are wounded

50. The epidermis is part of the:
    a. subcutaneous tissue
    b. muscle
    c. periosteum
    d. skin
    e. bone

51. Periosteum covers bone like fascia covers:
    a. skin
    b. fat
    c. muscle
    d. lung
    e. bladder

52. Subcutaneous tissue includes:
    a. skin
    b. connective tissue
    c. muscle
    d. fat
    e. b and d

53. Scar maturation occurs:
    a. as the last stage of tissue repair
    b. after all wounding including tattoos
    c. after the inflammatory stage
    d. all of the above
    e. none of the above

54. The only stage in which collagen fibers do not play a major role is:
    a. scar maturation
    b. proliferation and scar formation
    c. inflammation
    d. all of the above
    e. none of the above

55. Wound closure using sutures is termed:
    a. closure by primary intention
    b. closure by secondary intention
    c. granulation
    d. hemostasis
    e. none of the above

56. If during the course of an operation in which an initially clean wound was made and the pharyngeal cavity was entered, the wound is now:
    a. still a clean wound
    b. a contaminated wound
    c. a clean, contaminated wound
    d. an infected wound
    e. none of the above

57. "Dirty" wounds are:
    a. those which occur during sexual activity
    b. an already contaminated wound, for example, an abscess
    c. a wound which is initially clean but then the gastrointestinal tract is entered
    d. b and c

58. Factors which affect wound healing include:
    a. age
    b. steroids
    c. anti-neoplastic drugs
    d. weight
    e. all of the above

59. Factors which affect blood supply, and therefore wound healing, include:
    a. poor circulation secondary to cardiac dysfunction
    b. diabetes
    c. various vascular illnesses
    d. all of the above
    e. none of the above

60. Factors which affect wound healing include:
    a. chronic illness
    b. radiation therapy
    c. nutrition
    d. a and c
    e. all of the above

61. Complications seen in wound healing include:
    a. cellulitis
    b. scar maturation
    c. inflammation
    d. healing by tertiary intention
    e. none of the above

62. After primary closure about 95 percent of wound strength is reached by:
    a. six days
    b. six months
    c. six weeks
    d. four weeks
    e. fourteen days

63. Clean, contaminated wounds would include initially clean wounds which were then contaminated by:
    a. entrance into the pharyngeal cavity
    b. entrance into the genitourinary cavity
    c. entrance into the heart
    d. a and b
    e. none of the above

64. Contaminated wounds are also known as infected wounds. They are made through an already infected area where gross contamination by bacteria and/or other microorganisms are already present. We are giving you the answer so that you will not embarrass the authors by ever forgetting the definition of contaminated or infected wounds.

65. The method of wound closure during which the wound is only allowed to granulate closed is called:
    a. healing by primary intention
    b. healing by secondary intention
    c. healing by tertiary intention
    d. healing by quaternary intention
    e. none of the above

66. Hematomas usually result from:
    a. dehiscence of the wound
    b. cellulitis
    c. failure to obtain hemostasis at surgery
    d. a and b
    e. none of the above

67. Relaxed skin tension lines are:
    a. not important during surgery
    b. important for planning incisions
    c. the lines of minimal intention of the skin
    d. all of the above
    e. b and c

68. Areas of the wound that have not been adequately closed are called:
    a. dehiscences
    b. hematomas
    c. dead spaces
    d. seromas
    e. horrenudomas

69. Choice of suture material:
    a. is irrelevant
    b. depends upon the tissues and area of the body where the wound is to be closed
    c. is usually left up to the scrub nurse
    d. is whatever the hospital gives you
    e. all of the above

70. Basic principles in surgery include:
    a. relaxed skin tension lines
    b. incision planning
    c. tissue moisture
    d. hemostasis
    e. all of the above

71. Local anesthetics:
    a. prevent the sensation of pain
    b. work by blocking nerve conduction
    c. can be administered topically
    d. all of the above
    e. a and c

72. Which of the following is true?
    a. lidocaine's onset is immediate
    b. bupivacaine has a shorter duration than lidocaine
    c. procaine has a longer duration than bupivacaine
    d. the onset of action of all three is greater than five minutes
    e. all of the above

73. Which of the following is true?
    a. cocaine is a topical anesthetic
    b. lidocaine is both a topical and injectable anesthetic
    c. bupivacaine is primarily used as a vaso-constrictive agent
    d. a and b
    e. none of the above

74. The gauge of a needle refers to:
    a. its length
    b. the needle bore
    c. the needle diameter
    d. b and c
    e. none of the above

75. A wound under excessive postoperative stress can be caused by:
    a. exercise
    b. is not important in an adequately closed wound
    c. never contributes to seroma formation
    d. none of the above
    e. all of the above

76. Local anesthetics:
    a. are often used in combination with vaso-constrictive agents
    b. can reduce perioperative and postoperative pain
    c. can reduce the incidences of nausea and vomiting often associated with general anesthetics

    d. can facilitate earlier discharge from the hospital
    e. all of the above

77. Patients who are not good candidates for local anesthetics include:
    a. patients with a language barrier
    b. calm, cooperative patients
    c. anxious adults
    d. severely emotionally disturbed patients
    e. a, c and d

78. By Kern's rule, a 2% lidocaine solution has:
    a. 10 mg of drug per cc
    b. 20 mg of drug per cc
    c. 40 mg of drug per cc
    d. 80 mg of drug per cc
    e. none of the above

79. The reason a "test dose" is given when injecting local anesthetics is:
    a. since medical students are tortured so much, it is felt that everyone needs to be tested as much as possible
    b. to see if the drug will work
    c. to make sure no adverse reactions occur
    d. none of the above
    e. all of the above

80. Which of the following is true?
    a. the #10 blade is held at a 45-degree angle
    b. the #10 blade is held like a steak knife
    c. the #10 blade is held like a pencil
    d. the # 15 blade is held at a 30-degree angle
    e. a and c

81. The #10 blade is held:
    a. at a 30° angle
    b. like a steak knife
    c. at a 45° angle
    d. a and b
    e. b and c

82. The #15 blade is:
    a. larger than a #10 blade
    b. smaller than a #10 blade
    c. held at a 30° angle
    d. held like a steak knife
    e. not typically used for facial surgery

83. Tissue scissors:
    a. are also known as dissection scissors or undermining scissors
    b. are used to elevate or separate tissues
    c. usually have tips that are blunted
    d. a and c
    e. all of the above

N. 100 Quiz Questions

84. Needle holders come in several varieties, including:
   a. those with jaws with teeth
   b. those used for injection
   c. those without teeth
   d. a and c
   e. all of the above

85. The hemostat:
   a. can be either straight or curved
   b. can be used to dissect
   c. can be used as a needle holder
   d. should be held with the thumb and third finger in the ring holes
   e. a and b

86. A tail is left on a suture:
   a. for cosmetic purposes
   b. to give something that can be grasped to facilitate removal
   c. to prevent knot slippage, loosening, and undoing of the suture
   d. all of the above
   e. b and c

87. Electrocautery:
   a. is used for hemostasis
   b. comes in monopolar and bipolar forms
   c. works by using electrical current to coagulate blood vessels
   d. all of the above
   e. b and c

88. Monopolar cautery:
   a. generates less heat than bipolar
   b. can be used to cut tissues
   c. is usually used to cut skin
   d. transmits less heat to the surrounding tissue than bipolar cautery
   e. all of the above

89. A wound closure:
   a. can be facilitated by undermining of the skin surrounding the wound
   b. is rarely necessary
   c. should be done by closing anatomic layers
   d. a and c
   e. none of the above

90. A 6-0 suture is:
   a. larger diameter than a 4-0
   b. smaller diameter than a 4-0
   c. is too small for skin closure
   d. b and c
   e. none of the above

91. In children or noncompliant adults:
   a. absorbable suture is a good choice
   b. local anesthesia is a poor choice
   c. suture removal can be difficult in the case of children because of their failure to understand the need for it and their inherent fear of pain, and in the case of noncompliant adults because they may not show up for their follow-up appointment
   d. a and c
   e. all of the above

92. The two-hand tie:
   a. gives the best knot security
   b. is rarely used in surgery
   c. is not a tremendously useful tie
   d. b and c
   e. none of the above

93. In regard to suction devices:
   a. continuous suctions have a hole that can be plugged or unplugged
   b. intermittent suctions have a side port hole that should never be plugged
   c. suctions come in various types, including continuous suctions and intermittent suctions
   d. suctions are used to remove fluids from the field but should not be used to remove blood from the field due to risk of clotting off the suction
   e. on a continuous suction, when a side port hole is unplugged, the suction is turned off

94. The surgeon's knot:
   a. is the same as a square knot
   b. has two loops in the first throw
   c. is useful because the first throw with the two loops tends to stay in place better than the square knot
   d. b and c
   e. none of the above

95. Skin flaps can be used to:
   a. provide tissue coverage in wounds that have a tissue defect
   b. improve cosmetic results
   c. slow wound healing to an appropriate speed
   d. achieve homeostasis
   e. a and b

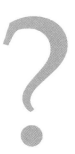

N. 100 Quiz Questions

96. The rotation flap:
    a. is appropriate for closing a circular defect
    b. is appropriate for closing a square defect
    c. is used to provide skin coverage when there is skin loss
    d. is appropriate for closing a triangular defect
    e. c and d

97. The Z-plasty:
    a. is useful in shortening wounds
    b. is useful in reorienting the direction of scars
    c. provides no improvement in cosmesis ever
    d. is a free flap
    e. is only used for closing square defects

98. Various types of skin flaps include:
    a. the advancement flap
    b. the rotation flap
    c. the trapezoid flap
    d. a and b
    e. all of the above

99. The Z-plasty, the rotation flap, and the advancement flap are all types of:
    a. local skin flaps
    b. complications of wound healing
    c. hypertrophic scars
    d. microvascular free flaps
    e. none of the above

100. The surgeon's knot:
    a. can be done as an instrument tie
    b. can be done as a two-hand tie
    c. can be done only by the surgeon
    d. b and c
    e. a and b

O. Glossary of Terms

anesthesiologist . . . .a physician specializing in administration of anesthetics

antineoplastic . . . . .inhibiting or preventing the development of cancer

bacteremia . . . . .the presence of bacteria in the blood

bevel . . . . .a slanting edge

biliary . . . . .relating to the system conveying bile

cardiopulmonary . . .pertaining to the heart and lungs

cellulitis . . . . .inflammation of the subcutaneous tissues

cicatrix . . . . .a scar; the new tissue formed in the healing of a wound

coagulation cascade . .sequence of chemical reactions that results in formation of a fibrin clot

collagen . . . . .the protein substance of connective tissues; part of scar formation in wound healing

debridement . . . . . . .the removal of foreign material

dehiscence . . . . .separation of the layers of a surgical wound; the falling apart of the wound

devitalized . . . . . . .to deprive of vitality or of life; the death of tissue

electrocardiogram . . .(ECG) a graphic tracing of the electrical activity of the heart muscle

electrolyte . . . . .a substance that dissociates into ions when in solution and is capable of conducting electricity; important elements in tissue fluids, like sodium, chloride, and potassium

endocrine . . . . .pertaining to internal secretions; hormonal; related to endocrine glands like thyroid, adrenal, pituitary, pancreas and thymus

enzyme . . . . .a protein molecule that speeds chemical reactions of other substances without being altered or destroyed itself

epinephrine . . . . . . .a vasoconstrictive agent that causes blood vessels to narrow or shrink down

erythematous . . . . . .redness of the skin

fibroblast . . . . .a connective tissue cell

gangrene . . . . .death of tissue due to a loss of vascular supply followed by infection

granulation tissue . .the formation of flesh masses, including new blood vessels, which appear in the wound during the healing process

hematoma . . . . .a collection of blood in an organ or tissue due to a break in the wall of a blood vessel; the swollen space that contains blood

hemostasis . . . . .interruption of the flow of blood through any vessel or to any anatomical area; stopping bleeding

HIV . . . . .human immunodeficiency virus; the virus that causes AIDS (acquired immunodeficiency syndrome)

hypertrophic scars . .hypertrophy; overgrowth and widening of scar tissue

immune . . . . .the body's protective response caused by injury or destruction of tissues

intubation . . . . .placement of a tube into a body canal or hollow organ, as into the trachea or stomach

O. Glossary of Terms

keloids . . . . .enlarged scars that extend beyond the limits of the original incision due to formation of excessive amounts of collagen

leukocytes . . . . .white blood cells

lymphocytes . . . . . . .white blood cells found in the blood, lymph, and lymphoid tissues

metabolic . . . . .all chemical changes that occur in living tissue

metabolism . . . . .the sum of all the physical and chemical processes by which living organisms maintain their function and survive

necrosis . . . . .tissue death

nurse anesthetist . . .a nurse (male or female) trained in the administration of anesthetics

oxygen saturation . . .the percent of oxygen bound to available hemoglobin

pathology . . . . .that branch of medicine which studies basic elements of disease, especially changes in the body caused by disease

perioperative . . . . . . .pertaining to the time period from the time of surgery to the time of discharge from the hospital

periosteum . . . . .thick tissue covering bone

postoperative . . . . . .time period occurring after a surgical operation

radiation therapy . . . . .treatment of cancers and other conditions with x-rays or any other appropriate rays

seroma . . . . .a collection of serum in the tissues

serum . . . . .body fluid, vascular fluid devoid of red blood cells

slough . . . . .shedding of dead tissue

sterile . . . . .the state of being aseptic or free of all microorganisms or spores

surgery . . . . .that branch of medicine which treats diseases, injuries and deformities by manual or operative methods

undermine . . . . .loosening and/or mobilizing tissue layers by using a scalpel or scissors

vasoconstrictive . . . .characterized by a decrease in the diameter of a blood vessel; to narrow or shrink down blood vessels

viscera . . . . .internal organs located inside the body cavity

P. 100 Quiz Answers

1. c	21. a	41. a	61. a	81. d
2. a	22. b	42. c	62. c	82. b
3. d	23. c	43. c	63. d	83. e
4. b	24. b	44. e	64. free	84. d
5. a	25. e	45. e	65. b	85. e
6. a	26. d	46. a	66. c	86. e
7. b	27. d	47. e	67. e	87. d
8. c	28. e	48. a	68. c	88. b
9. b	29. e	49. e	69. b	89. d
10. d	30. e	50. d	70. e	90. b
11. b	31. e	51. c	71. d	91. e
12. c	32. e	52. e	72. a	92. a
13. a	33. a	53. d	73. d	93. c
14. e	34. d	54. c	74. d	94. d
15. a	35. d	55. a	75. a	95. e
16. c	36. b	56. c	76. e	96. e
17. b	37. c	57. b	77. e	97. b
18. e	38. c	58. e	78. b	98. d
19. e	39. e	59. d	79. c	99. a
20. e	40. b	60. e	80. b	100. e

Fill in the number of *your* correct answers. _____

Index

Note: Page numbers followed by f refer to figures; page numbers followed by t refer to tables.

Q. Main Menu for CD ROM (Disc 1)

 CD-ROM icon indicates supplemental audio-visual materials
that can be seen on the CD.

1. **Scrubbing - washing hands**
2. **Gowning and Gloving**
3. **Surgical Instruments**
   a. *Scalpel*
   b. *Tissue Scissors*
   c. *Forceps*
   d. *Skin Hooks*
   e. *Retractor*
   f. *Needle Holder (Needle Driver)*
   g. *Hemostat*
   h. *Suction*
   i. *Cautery*
   j. *Needle Driver*
   k. *Suture Scissors*
   l. *Towel Clip*
   m. *Staple Gun*
   n. *Endoscopic Equipment*
4. **Knot Tying - (Right Handed) Video Animation**
   a. *Two Hand Tie*
      1. *Square Knot*
      2. *Surgeon's Knot*
      3. *Comparison Between Surgeon's Knot and Square Knot*
   b. *Instrument Tie*

5. **Knot Tying - (Left Handed) Video Animation**
   a. *Two Hand Tie*
      1. *Square Knot*
      2. *Surgeon's Knot*
      3. *Comparison Between Surgeon's Knot and Square Knot*
   b. *Instrument Tie*
6. **Endoscopic Tying**

R. Main Menu for CD ROM (Disc 2)

1. **Laboratory Preparations (Pigs' Feet)**
2. **Laboratory Exercises (Surgical Techniques)**
   a. *Instructions and Directions*
      1. *Making an incicision*
      2. *Undermining*
      3. *Principle of Halving*
   b. *Closing of Skin*
      1. *Suture Techniques*
         a. *Simple Interrupted Suture*
         b. *Vertical Mattress*
         c. *Horizontal Mattress*
         d. *Running Closure ("Baseball Stitch")*
         e. *Running-Lock Closure*
         f. *Running Intracuticular Closure*
         g. *Staple Closure*
         h. *Endoscopic Suturing*
      2. *Skin Adhesive Closure - Dermabond®*
   c. *Skin Flaps*
      1. *Fusiform Excision*
      2. *Advancement Flap*
      3. *Rotation Flap*
      4. *Z-Plasty*
      5. *Note Flap*
      6. *Bilobe Flap*
      7. *Rhombic Flap*
      8. *W-Plasty*
      9. *Geometric Broken Line Closure*
      10. *4 Examples of Local Flaps in Patients*

3. **Quiz**
   a. **All 101 questions with answers — immediate feed back, answers scored.**
   b. **25 randomized questions without answers, scored after conclusion of quiz.**

S. Notes from CD ROM

S. Notes from CD ROM

T. Acknowledgments

To all those who made this work possible we say thank you and that includes the creative production team at Mayo Clinic, Thomas E. Bibby, Lizabeth D. Daube, George DeVinny, Melissa C. Freetly, Fred Graszer, David M. Jorgenson, Joseph M. Kane, Mark J. McGlinch, Kurt J. Simon; the artists, David A. Factor, M. Alice McKinney, and James D. Postier; our loyal and professional operating room staff, Ann D. Archer, James D. Clark, Linda A. Fenske, Barbara C. Griffith, Karman L. McGill, Barbara K. Pehler-Williams, and Denise K. Webbles; our secretaries, Michelle T. Franke, Kelly Amunrud, Denise Rogers, Tracy Tollefson, and Brenda J. Prondzinski; and two of our residents Nissim Khabie, M.D. and Matthew A. Kienstra, M.D.; and two of our medical students Darren McDonald and Natalie Strand. We thank you all for your superior advice and constructive criticisms which made this work the quality that it is today; finally, a very giant thank you and most grateful appreciation to our chair, Thomas J. McDonald, M.D. for his more than generous support of this project.

David A. Sherris, M.D.
Eugene B. Kern, M.D.
2004

U. Instructions for CD ROM Installation

To install Essential Surgical Skills

Note: If the program is installed on your hard drive, the CD must be in the drive when running the program

Windows 95/98/NT

1. Insert the Essential Surgical Skills CD ROM in your CD-ROM drive.
2. After Essential Surgical Skills starts, quit the program.
3. Go to your computer **Start** menu on the task bar. Select **Run**.
4. Type D:\setup.exe (or E:\setup.exe if your CD Drive is E:) and press **Enter.**
5. Follow the on-screen instructions.
6. The installation program will make a Surgical Skills item in your **Programs** menu

Macintosh

1. Insert the Essential Surgical Skills CD ROM in your CD-ROM drive.
2. Create a folder on your hard drive named "Essential Surgical Skills"
3. Copy the following items to the new folder you just created.
   Surgical Skills
   Xtras folder
   QuickTime Overlay
4. Double-click **Surgical Skills** icon to start the program.

V. Operating CD ROM

To run the program from the CD ROM

Windows 95/98/NT

1. Insert the *Essential Surgical Skills* CD ROM in your CD ROM drive.

2. If *Essential Surgical Skills* does not begin automatically, go to your computer **Start** menu on the task bar. Select **Run**.

3. Type D:\SurgicalSkills.exe (or E:\SurgicalSkills.exe if your CD Drive is E:) and press **Enter**.

Macintosh

1. Insert the *Essential Surgical Skills* CD ROM in your CD ROM drive.

2. Double-click the **Surgical Skills** icon.

Note: To view the Essential Surgical Skills at full screen, change your monitor resolution to 1024x768. See your computer documentation for instructions.

Minimum System Requirements

Windows 95/98/NT

CD-ROM drive:	4x speed
Computer Processor:	486/90 or faster processor
Memory:	16 MB of RAM
Operation System:	Windows 95, Windows 98, or Windows NT 3.51 or 4.0
Hard Disk space:	15MB of disk space
Video:	Compatible SGVA Card
Sound:	Soundblaster compatible sound card
Video for Windows	

Macintosh

Minimum System requirements:

CD-ROM drive:	4x speed
Computer Processor:	Power PC 66
Memory:	12 MB of RAM
Operation System:	System 7.51
Hard Disk space:	15MB of disk space
Video:	Supports thousands/millions of colors
QuickTime 2 or better	